# Respectful Relationships in the Maternity Service

Maggie O'Brien · Ellen Kitson-Reynolds

**Editors**

# Respectful Relationships in the Maternity Service

## A Guide to Achieving a Positive Midwifery Culture

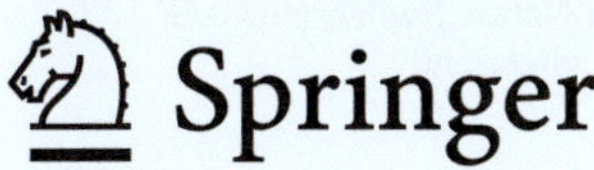

*Editors*
Maggie O'Brien
University of Southampton
Southampton, United Kingdom

Ellen Kitson-Reynolds
University of Southampton
Southampton, United Kingdom

Royal College of Midwives RCMF (Hons)
London, United Kingdom

Editorial Contact: Marie-Elia Come-Garry

ISBN 978-3-032-04280-4      ISBN 978-3-032-04281-1   (eBook)
https://doi.org/10.1007/978-3-032-04281-1

*To my midwife friends and colleagues who have walked beside me for part or all of this incredible midwifery journey*

*To Paul, Stacey and Riley who together have proven that anything is possible*

# Preface

The driver for writing this book originates from representing midwives as a Royal College of Midwives regional officer, witnessing the distress and physical and mental health symptoms of midwives who had been treated disrespectfully in their workplace. Some of these midwives left midwifery altogether and suffered serious long-term health effects. Later, in Director of Midwifery roles I quickly realised that when cultures are unkind and hierarchical a few individuals are 'permitted' to abuse power; resulting in others changing their behaviour to 'fit in'. Having developed a desire to create innovative, kind cultures where everyone is valued it became essential to develop

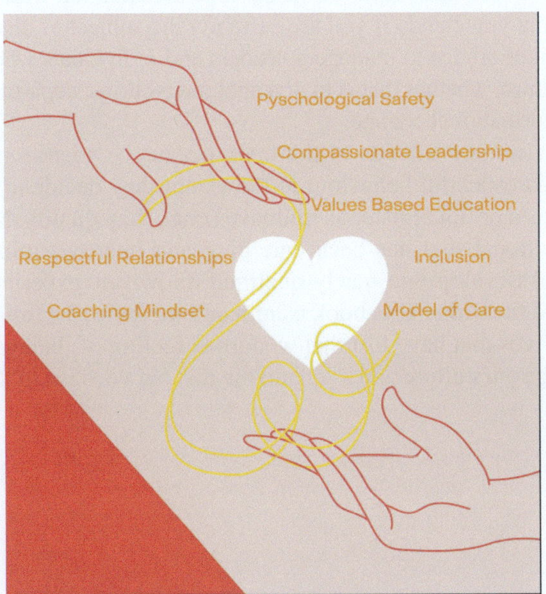


The 'Golden Threads of Change'. (Courtesy of Maggie O'Brien and Yvonne O'Doherty)

---

The original version of the book has been revised. The correction to this book can be found at https://doi.org/10.1007/978-3-032-04281-1_9

strategies for culture change. Some of these strategies proved transformational and some were not so successful; but important lessons were learnt along the way. Some of the vignettes, examples and case studies provided in this book are taken from all the authors' experiences of culture change and some are taken from examples given by compassionate, inspirational leaders, proven successful in achieving culture change.

Research and reviews of maternity services over many years have proven that maternity and neonatal cultures are sometimes unkind and psychologically unsafe. This results in women and birthing people, maternity staff and student midwives being subjected to disrespectful behaviour including, in some instances, bullying. The consequences of this are that some maternity unit staff are scared to speak up, causing these maternity units to become increasingly unsafe, with high sickness and turnover rates among midwives and a high dropout rate among student midwives. As the writing of the chapters evolved and on speaking to a wide range of leaders from all four countries of the United Kingdom, several 'golden threads' emerged, identified by the authors as essential to culture change. These 'golden threads' are achieving respectful relationships, compassionate leadership, a coaching mindset, inclusion, psychological safety and a compassionate model of care, including ways of working. The book explores the evidence that disrespectful behaviour has existed for many years, explaining the difference between disrespectful and bullying behaviours, including the detrimental effects of both. The evidence that maternity and neonatal units are currently under intense pressure, what the stressors are and how they impact on behaviour is examined and discussed. However, the main focus of the book is on resolution with advice and guidance given on what you can do if you are currently the subject of disrespectful behaviour. It also provides advice to managers, leaders and individuals who want to change their working culture, whether that is in personal interactions, departmental changes or whole unit transformational change.

Student midwives are a focus of the book because evidence suggests they are also subject to disrespectful behaviour to the extent they decide to leave their midwifery programmes or not register as midwives once they qualify. More recently, as a midwife educationalist it has been enriching and heart-warming to experience student midwives develop into newly qualified midwives, experiencing the joy of midwifery for the first time. This book is intended for them, the future of midwifery, and for all midwives that have lost that wondrous feeling of 'being a midwife'; it is possible to change our culture and to regain the joy, but we have to do it together and with kindness.

West Sussex, UK                                                                       Maggie O'Brien

# Acknowledgements

A heartfelt thank you to everyone that has made the completion of this book possible. To Ellen who agreed to write a chapter and edit the book with me, whose wisdom and patience has known no bounds and without who I would never of realized my dream.

To all of the contributing authors, Lesley, Jennifer, Marie, Helen, Denise and Emer for writing their chapters, and providing encouragement, expertise and knowledge, thank you does not seem enough.

To Yvonne O'Doherty, thank you for your understanding of what was required and your artwork and patience.

To Emma Batt an ex-Maternity Voices Chair who gave me some great insights into how women and birthing people perceive compassionate midwifery care.

To Amanda Burleigh, RM, RGN, BSc. Hons, who helped me with the detail around the Say no to Bullying in Midwifery Facebook page and who has done a huge amount to support midwives and student midwives who have been bullied.

To the inspirational leaders who agreed to speak to me, a special thank you for the enlightening conversations on how they display compassion and how they achieved and maintained culture change. These leaders are:

Dr Mary Ross-Davie,
Director of Midwifery,
NHS Greater Glasgow and Clyde

Carla Jones,
Director of Midwifery,
University Hospital Birmingham

Jaki Lambert Director,
Royal College Midwives,
Scotland

Nicola McGovern,
Community Midwifery Manager,
James Paget University Hospitals, NHS Trust

Jess Read
Midwife, Leadership Coach

Jeanne Tarrant,
Fitness to Practice Officer,
Nursing and Midwifery Board of Ireland

Gill Walton CBE
CEO, Royal College of Midwives

Finally thank you to Springer Nature, in particular Marie-Elia Comme-Garry for her belief and encouragement and Shirly Christina for her endless patience.

# Contents

# Editors and Contributors

## About the Editors

**Maggie O'Brien**   Maggie has held senior midwifery leadership positions both in the UK and New Zealand, including the Director of Midwifery for Imperial College NHS Trust and for Auckland District Health Board. She has had experience of cultural change in both countries and believes strongly in the importance of developing compassionate cultures for women and midwives. Her most recent role was Senior Teaching Fellow at the University of Southampton and believes it essential to provide supportive environments for student midwives, enabling them to reach their full potential.

She was elected President of the Royal College of Midwives from 2004 until 2008 and received an Honorary Fellowship from the RCM in 2009.

**Dr. Ellen Kitson-Reynolds**   Ellen is Deputy Head of School for Education, Principal Teaching Fellow and Principal Fellow—HEA, at the University of Southampton. Her interests link to transition from student to qualified practitioner, clinical decision making and autonomous practice, continuity of carer, interprofessional education and bladder management.

## About the Contributors

**Emer Kelly**   Emer is a Senior Teaching Fellow in Midwifery at the University of Southampton. Her background is in Nursing (Women's Health Promotion) and high-risk midwifery care in her previous role as a Clinical Midwifery Manager. She is passionate about women's psychological well-being during pregnancy, intrapartum and postpartum. She leads on the modules for Obstetric Emergencies and Enhanced Postpartum Care, including the Newborn Infant and Physical Examination. She continues to work clinically and ensures her updated practice is reflected in her teaching. She is equally passionate about student support and is a Schwartz Round facilitator for healthcare students within the university.

**Jennifer Lancaster**   Jennifer is a Senior Teaching Fellow at the University of Southampton. With a background of study in Psychology with Sociology and Performance Psychology, and previous clinical roles within Maternity Practice

Education and as Midwifery Preceptorship Programme Lead, she is passionate about supporting a safe working environment and preparing student midwives for a successful transition to autonomous practitioners.

**Denise Linay**   Denise has had a long and varied career in midwifery, beginning in clinical practice before moving to the Royal College of Midwives. There, she held roles as a Regional Officer and Employment Relations Advisor before becoming Head of Organising and Engagement, a position she held from 2012 until her retirement in 2020.

In 2019, she qualified as a Professional Coach and now works as a Career and Leadership Coach. She is currently pursuing a master's in Coaching at Warwick University. In 2022, she co-founded Coaches in Mind with Helen Rogers.

Her interests include weightlifting, running, hiking, theatre, reading, writing and travel. She also writes a personal blog, 60 is the New 60.

**Dr. Marie Naish**   Marie is a Senior Teaching Fellow at the University of Southampton. Her roles and responsibilities at the University include Lead Midwife for Education, Midwifery Programme Lead and Group Manager. Her clinical background includes continuity of care midwifery practice, providing care to women and families aged 18 and under across the childbirth continuum. Her interests include equality, diversity and inclusion, and she is passionate about reducing health inequalities. In 2025, she completed her doctoral study exploring the experiences of women, birth partners and midwives of a dedicated, 24-hour, telephone support line for labour.

**Helen Rogers**   Helen's background is in health. She trained as a nurse before going on to qualify as a midwife in the UK. She then left a clinical career to join the Royal College of Midwives, first as a Regional Officer and then as Director for Wales. She has always had an interest in coaching and has been lucky to have a senior leadership role that has enabled her to coach on an informal level for most of her career. She believes that coaching can and does make a huge difference in terms of an individual's confidence, performance and contribution to the organisation that they work in. Having qualified as a Professional Coach in 2017, she now provides leadership and career coaching to clients primarily, but not exclusively, from the NHS and maternity services. She is the co-founder, with Denise Linay, of Coaches in Mind. Her interests include gardening, sewing, quilting, running, yoga, reading and walking.

**Dr. Lesley Turner**   Lesley is a Senior Teaching Fellow in Midwifery and Head of Practice Education at the University of Southampton. She is invested in improving the learning environment for students and has recently shared processes for students to raise concerns relating to their support and assessment in clinical areas.

In her research role, she has been working on quantitative research on the association between staffing levels and the quality of midwifery care including postnatal experience, readmission rates and adverse events.

# Abbreviations

| | |
|---|---|
| ACAS | Advisory Conciliatory Arbitration Service |
| ADHD | Attention Deficit Hyperactivity Disorder |
| ASD | Autism Spectrum Disorder |
| AI | Artificial Intelligence |
| AIMS | Association of Improvement in Maternity Services |
| ARMS | Association of Radical Midwives |
| AC | Association for Coaching |
| ALS | Action Learning Sets |
| BMM | Black Maternity Matters |
| CNO | Chief Nursing Officer |
| CTG | Cardiotocograph |
| CQC | Care Quality Commission |
| DH | Department of Health |
| DHSC | Department of Health and Social Security |
| DOM | Director of Midwifery |
| DON | Director of Nursing |
| DSA | Disabled Student Allowance |
| EDIB | Equity, Diversity Inclusion Belonging |
| FTE | Full Time Equivalent |
| GP | General Practitioner |
| HCC | Health Care Commission |
| HEI | Higher Education Institution |
| HOM | Head of Midwifery |
| HR | Human Resources |
| ICC | International Coaching Confederation |
| ICU | Intensive Care Unit |
| IPA | Interpretive Phenomenological Analysis |
| IPE | Interprofessional Education |
| LMC | Lead Maternity Carer |
| MBRRACE-UK | Mother Baby Reducing Risk through Audits Confidential Enquires-United Kingdom |
| MECC | Make Every Contact Count |
| MCC | Master Certified Coach |
| MLDP | Midwifery Leadership and Development Programme |

| | |
|---|---|
| MSF | Manufacturing Science Finance (Trade Union) |
| MSLC | Maternity Services Liaison Committee |
| MSW | Maternity Support Worker |
| NCT | National Childbirth Trust |
| NHS | National Health Service |
| NHSE | NHS England |
| NMC | Nursing and Midwifery Council |
| NZ | New Zealand |
| OED | *Oxford English Dictionary* |
| PMA | Professional Midwifery Advocate |
| PPE | Personal Protective Equipment |
| RePAIR | Reducing Pre-registration Attrition and Improving Retention |
| RCM | Royal College of Midwives |
| RCN | Royal College of Nursing |
| TRiM | Trauma Risk Management |
| TUC | Trade Union Congress |
| UK | United Kingdom |
| UNISON | Refers to the union of public service workers itself |
| VBE | Values-Based Education |
| VUCA | Volatile Unsafe Complex Ambitious |
| WHO | World Health Organisation |

# List of Boxes

# Introduction

**1**

Maggie O'Brien

## 1.1 Introduction

This book provides a guide on how to achieve culture change by drawing on research evidence and compassionate leader's experiences of successfully changing maternity culture. You may be asking yourself why a book focusing on achieving positive maternity and neonatal culture is necessary, particularly as birth is usually one of the most joyful, positive experiences that anyone has the privilege to witness. Without doubt (speaking from experience), midwifery is one of the most wondrous, fulfilling professions to enter, with many inspirational and nurturing midwives providing safe, high-quality midwifery care to women and birthing people. Therefore, it is sad and demoralising that disrespectful cultures have evolved in some maternity and neonatal units across the United Kingdom (UK), creating distress and disillusionment for some of the women and birthing people we care for and the staff working within them. Students are crucial to the future of midwifery and the maternity workforce, but are sometimes impacted by unkind, insensitive behaviour; therefore, improving students experience is one focus of this book.

One of the intentions of the authors is to give hope and a belief to all midwives, student midwives, maternity and neonatal staff and managers, who find themselves, through no fault of their own, working in unkind, disrespectful cultures, that change is achievable. Through providing vignettes, case studies and examples of how compassionate leaders have successfully changed culture, the author's intention is to give people courage to take the first steps towards change. To be kind to women and birthing people and to work colleagues is a professional requirement (Nursing and Midwifery Council [NMC] 2019) and integral to the role of all staff working within maternity and neonatal services, with most maternity and neonatal staff providing

M. O'Brien (✉)
University of Southampton, Southampton, United Kingdom

Royal College of Midwives RCMF (Hons), London, United Kingdom
e-mail: Mahues935@gmail.com



M. O'Brien, E. Kitson-Reynolds (eds.), *Respectful Relationships in the Maternity Service*, https://doi.org/10.1007/978-3-032-04281-1_1

1

kind, compassionate and high-quality care. However, indisputable national and international research evidence spanning many years (Burleigh et al. 2023; Capper et al. 2022; Catling and Rossiter 2020; Catling et al. 2017; Royal College of Midwives [RCM] 1996, 2016; Gillen et al. 2008; Ball et al. 2002; Hadikin and O'Driscoll 2000), together with repeated findings of maternity services reviews (Care Quality Commission [CQC] 2024; Independent Maternity Review 2022; Kirkup 2015, 2022; Francis 2013; Commission for Healthcare Audit and Inspection 2006), demonstrates that kindness and compassion are not always central to care provided by some National Health Service (NHS) Trusts to women and birthing people, their families and the staff working within them. The lack of kindness and compassion is encapsulated by Donna Ockenden in her initial report, *Report of emerging themes of the Independent Maternity Review at the Shrewsbury and Telford Hospital NHS Trust.*

> One of the most disappointing and deeply worrying themes that has emerged is the reported lack of kindness and compassion from some members of the maternity team at the Trust. Healthcare professionals are in a privileged position caring for women and their families at a pivotal time on their lives. Many of the cases reviewed have tragic outcomes where kindness and compassion is even more essential. The fact that this had found to be lacking on many occasions is unacceptable and deeply concerning. (Ockenden 2020, p. 11, 4.3)

## 1.2   Who Will Benefit from Reading This Book?

The practical guidance provided will benefit individuals who are being, or have been, subjected to disrespectful behaviour, or are in the process of changing a clinical or educational workplace culture. The research evidence, case studies and vignettes presented focus on maternity and neonatal services and midwifery, mainly in the UK; however, non-compassion within maternity and neonatal services is a universal issue (Mayra et al. 2023; Capper et al. 2022; Catling et al. 2017; Catling and Rossiter 2020), meaning that a guide to achieving positive cultures will be beneficial to staff working in healthcare environments worldwide. Mayra et al. (2023) discuss maternity care in India and Nigeria, arguing that compassion *for* midwives is essential for compassion to be provided *by* midwives, a concept explored within this book, including how this is possible to achieve. Given that many members of staff working within the National Health Service (NHS) are currently working in negative cultures and suffering the detrimental effects (Darzi 2024; Burleigh et al. 2023; Kirkup 2022), *all* maternity and neonatal staff, including midwives, student midwives, doctors, student doctors, nurses, student nurses, neonatal nurses and maternity support workers (MSW) would benefit from the practical advice and encouragement provided by the authors of this book. In addition to NHS staff, advice given will benefit healthcare staff providing care in the private, voluntary and independent sectors. There is published research evidence that student midwives are sometimes subject to disrespectful behaviour in clinical practice and/or whilst at university both within the UK and internationally (McNeil and Kitson-Reynolds 2024; Wylam 2023; Capper 2021; Oates et al. 2020; Johnston 2016; Kitson-Reynolds 2010; Gillen et al. 2008, 2009; Begley 2002), making the advice given within this book a valuable resource for students and educationalists situated in universities, NHS Trusts, the public, voluntary or independent sectors and international health services.

## 1.3 What Is the Purpose of This Book?

The purpose of the book is to draw together evidence and compassionate leader's experiences to provide a guide for maternity and neonatal staff and students on how to achieve positive cultures in their workplaces. This may be by making small changes within a working relationship, a department or a transformational change involving a whole maternity and/or neonatal service. The purpose of achieving positive maternity and neonatal cultures is for *all* staff to feel respected, valued, supported and included, resulting in improved safety, quality of care and increased kindness to women and birthing people and neonates. The authors provide guidance on how psychologically safe cultures can be achieved, where zero tolerance of disrespectful behaviour exists; until we achieve this, maternity and neonatal staff currently providing kind and compassionate care will continue to feel demoralised every time the findings of a maternity services review is made public, with disrespectful and bullying behaviours continuing to thrive unchallenged.

Research proves that disrespectful and bullying behaviours exist (see Sect. 2.2), causing significant mental and physical harm to maternity and neonatal staff (see Sect. 2.7.3). This book provides guidance on *how* to achieve respectful relationships and positive workplace cultures, with the aim of preventing disrespectful and bullying behaviours. It provides examples of culture change, practical advice, case studies and vignettes from compassionate leaders, who have successfully changed the culture of their workplaces and learnt valuable lessons whilst doing so. The second chapter provides a background and context to the book, whilst the third chapter explores the intense pressures that maternity and neonatal staff are currently experiencing (Smith 2021) that can sometimes be the reason for staff displaying unacceptable behaviour. Chapters 4, 5, 6, and 7 consider values-based education (VBE), developing a coaching mindset, implementation of Schwartz Rounds and compassionate leadership as ways of achieving change culture. It should be emphasised that to change a disrespectful culture is not an easy task and sometimes change has been attempted with limited success, but important lessons have been learnt along the way. The authors do not pretend to have all the answers, but if we *all* make small changes, anything is possible, provided we continue to *dare to dream*, as described by Jan Smith (2021) in the final chapter of her excellent book *Nurturing Maternity Staff* (Smith 2021).

## 1.4　Language Used to Describe Behaviours

Much thought and debate occurred when deciding the title of this book, some believing that the word *bullying* should be included in the title, whilst others thought that this would be demoralising for staff and students working within maternity and neonatal services. Eventually, a decision was made by the authors not to use the term *bullying* because it is believed that very few midwives, maternity and neonatal staff are actual bullies. Most people who display disrespectful behaviour do so because of many possible stressors, including inadequate staffing levels, lack of physiological safety and working within disrespectful cultures; it was, therefore, decided to use the terminology *respectful relationships* in the title and *disrespectful behaviour* throughout the book to take account of these factors. This was agreed by the authors with the caveat that an acknowledgement of the fact that bullying behaviour is sometimes at the centre of disrespectful cultures and can cause long-term, devastating effects on maternity and neonatal staff. It is important to understand the difference between disrespectful behaviour and bullying and use correct terminology when addressing unacceptable workplace behaviours (see Sect. 2.6). Where the term *bullying* is used, it is to cite other authors, discuss published research, books and articles that explore and refer to bullying behaviour and when discussing how incidents involving bullying behaviour can be identified and resolved.

In acknowledgement of gender-diverse people and people whose gender identity does not align with the sex they were assigned at birth, the term *women and birthing people* is used throughout the book, except occasionally, where the term *service user* is used in the wider context of coaching and user representation.

## 1.5　What Does the Book Have to Offer?

The authors identify, explore and discuss factors essential for achieving positive maternity and neonatal cultures. These factors are described as 'golden threads of change'; the Oxford English Dictionary (OED) describes golden threads as 'an idea or feature that is present in all parts of something, holds it together and gives it value' (OED 2025). The 'golden thread' philosophy originated in Greek mythology with Theseus, who followed a golden thread given to him by Ariadne to find his way out of the Minotaur's cave (Mills and Reeve 2021). In 2018, NHS England (NHSE) envisaged the concept of the golden thread of safety running through healthcare as a catalyst for the change required (NHSE 2018). As the writing of this book progressed, essential factors emerged as 'golden threads', which are believed crucial to achieving *safe*, positive, respectful maternity and neonatal cultures. It became clear that the 'golden threads' are interlinked and, when woven together, are transformational in changing negative, disrespectful cultures into positive, respectful ones. The 'golden threads of change' that emerged are respectful relationships, inclusion, developing a coaching mindset, providing values-based education, compassionate models of care, compassionate leadership, and achieving psychological safety (see

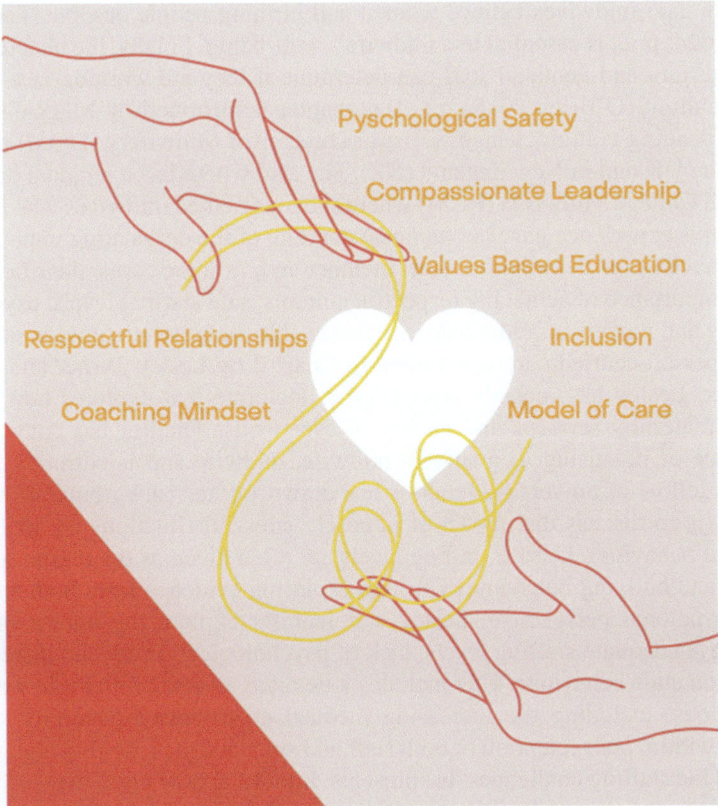


**Fig. 1.1** The 'Golden Threads of Change'. (Courtesy of Maggie O'Brien and Yvonne Doherty)

Fig. 1.1). The final chapter weaves the 'golden threads of change' together with experiences of compassionate leaders to give guidance on how change is possible.

Chapter 2 begins by asking the question, 'how have we arrived at a position where the findings of every maternity service review (Kirkup 2015, 2022; Independent Maternity Review 2022) identify a lack of kindness and compassion to women and birthing people and maternity staff?' Maggie O'Brien provides a background and context to the book by exploring research evidence and reviews of maternity services to determine 'how did we get here?' Maggie goes on to describe how both positive and negative cultures develop and flourish, identifies the differences between disrespectful and bullying behaviour, explaining the physiological, psychological and behavioural harm these behaviours cause to women and birthing people, maternity, neonatal staff and their families (O'Brien 2018b). The importance of kindness and compassion is explored through the lens of women and birthing people, with an emphasis on how an equitable, diverse, inclusive and belonging (EDIB) culture is more likely to be empathetic and compassionate (West 2021). The chapter discusses the provision of compassionate models of care, explaining that providing care midwives believe women and birthing people deserve (Feeley and Stacey 2024, p. 2) is essential to a midwife's well-being. Finally, the chapter details how maternity and neonatal staff can determine if they are working in a compassionate culture (O'Brien 2018a, c). The chapter is informed by Maggie's experiences of leading culture change whilst in Director of Midwifery (DOM) positions both in the UK and in New Zealand (NZ). She also worked as a regional officer for the Royal College Midwives (RCM) where she represented midwives who had been bullied; this experience gave her an understanding of the devastating impact of bullying behaviour on an individual staff member and, in some cases, their families.

The importance of achieving respectful cultures, safe staffing levels, psychological safety and models of midwifery care that enable midwives to provide safe, high-quality, person-centred care is explored in Chap. 3 by Lesley Turner and Jennifer Lancaster. Lesley has recently completed a doctorate that explores how staffing impacts maternity services and quality of care whilst Jennifer has contemporary experience of practising as a student midwife, midwife and is currently a senior teaching fellow at university. Jennifer has drawn on her background of studying psychology to discuss the impact of intensely stressful situations on staff's well-being and behaviour. Unsafe staffing levels are often given as the reason for disrespectful and bullying behaviour. Through exploring evidence from both a national and international perspective, Lesley and Jennifer explore the impact of stress, including inadequate staffing levels, lack of psychological safety and disrespectful cultures on staff behaviour. This includes a detailed review of multiple workplace complexities, including the increasing medical environment maternity staff are working within, poor retention of both staff and students, the resulting high vacancy rates and the staffing challenges this presents. It looks at how midwives can become vulnerable to these complexities, resulting in work-related stress, burnout and psychological ill-health. The culture and impact of coping are discussed where the continual low staffing levels and challenging situations are normalised, with an expectation that staff will be 'resilient' and cope *no matter what*.

Ellen-Kitson Reynolds and Marie Naish begin Chap. 4 by stating that the future of midwifery rests with our students and asks if students, educators and clinicians can meet the challenge this presents. Whilst written primarily for student midwives, Chap. 4 provides an inspiration for newly qualified midwives, practice supervisors and assessors, practice education teams and midwifery educators. It gives readers of the book an understanding of compassion, empathy and emotional intelligence, illustrating how they promote a compassionate and kind culture within midwifery practice. The chapter will help you to find and realise your strengths and to develop professionally from them. Ellen is currently Deputy Head of School for Education, and her doctorate research focused on the transition from being a student midwife to becoming a newly qualified practitioner (Kitson-Reynolds 2010). Marie has recently completed a doctorate and is currently Midwifery Programme Lead; both use their experience of creating, validating and implementing a values-based curriculum (Kitson-Reynolds 2020) to present and consider how the experiences of students can be improved through their education. Throughout the chapter, Ellen and Marie ask students to apply concepts to their real-world experiences of midwifery education and to forward project and consider how this could impact their future career and care provision, asking whether they are up to the task of supporting future learners in both their student role and as a newly qualified midwife.

Helen Rogers and Denise Linay identify developing a coaching mindset as a 'golden thread of change' (OED 2025) in Chap. 5, where the promotion and use of coaching are reinforced as a key element of cultural change, identifying how a genuine coaching mindset can be transformational when it becomes established practice for all employees. Helen and Denise dispel the assumption that coaching is just for senior leaders; instead, showing how a coaching mindset approach can be used in different settings and with staff who are in any position within an organisation. Helen and Denise are founders of Coaching in Mind (2025), whose mission is 'to support healthcare professionals to maximise their potential. To be the authentic, dynamic and compassionate professionals they aspire to be' (Rogers and Linay 2025). They both use their extensive experience, gained by having held senior positions within the RCM and as qualified coaches, to describe what coaching is but also what it isn't. They then move on to look at the skills you as an individual will need if you wish to develop a coaching mindset, have successful coaching conversations and enhance a coaching approach within your workplace. Case studies and vignettes are used to demonstrate how powerful and transformational a coaching conversation can be. Following this, the chapter explores the history of coaching in the NHS, asking what, if any, embedding has taken place and asks if what is provided is really coaching. Helen and Denise conclude with the impact coaching can have, explaining what a ripple effect is and how powerful and effective it can be in creating strong supportive cultures.

Schwartz Rounds are described in Chap. 6 as powerful catalysts for achieving positive maternity and neonatal culture change (Maben et al. 2021). As an experienced midwife in providing high-risk care, Emer Kelly has acquired a knowledge and awareness of the impact of providing care in a high-risk setting on the wellbeing of midwives and student midwives. Now a Senior Teaching Fellow, she is passionate about supporting students and, as such, is a Schwartz Round facilitator for university students. Schwartz Rounds are described as confidential, reflective forums that enable both maternity and neonatal staff and students to consider the rewards and challenges of working in clinical practice (The Point of Care Foundation 2025). Emer explains that reflection can provide improvements in care to women and birthing people, which can lead to staff engagement and enhancement of wellbeing. Schwartz Rounds foster psychological safety to encourage all attendees to reflect on the emotional aspects of their work (The Point of Care Foundation 2025). Schwartz Rounds provide a non-judgemental way to provide support to all, reinforcing our values, reminding us why we chose our profession and restoring commitment to compassionate care.

The importance of implementing compassionate leadership to achieve culture change in maternity and neonatal services is explored by Maggie O'Brien in Chap. 7. The compassionate leadership approach, developed by Professor Michael West over the last few years, is described as understanding and applying the four elements of compassion: *attending*, *understanding*, *empathising* and *helping* to the context of leading others (West 2021; West and Bailey 2022; West and Chowla 2017; West et al. 2017). Different perspectives are then drawn together to visualise compassionate leadership through a range of lenses. First, it asks what *you* think compassionate leadership is, and then it considers what *we* think compassionate leadership is, going on to challenge the myth that compassionate leadership is weak leadership. The end of the chapter draws together the views of compassionate leaders of maternity services, who have successfully implemented culture change within their organisations, exploring the qualities essential for compassionate leaders and the actions they have taken to demonstrate compassionate leadership. All leaders identified compassionate leadership as crucial to culture change and as such, it is identified as one of the 'golden threads of change' (OED 2025).

In the final chapter, 'Finding Resolution', Maggie O'Brien weaves the 'golden threads of change' together with her experiences of culture change and those of compassionate leaders to provide examples and guidance on how to achieve positive maternity cultures. Maggie explores respectful relationships, inclusion, values-based education, a coaching mindset, compassionate models of midwifery care, compassionate leadership and psychological safety as a framework for transforming negative maternity and neonatal cultures to nurturing, kind and compassionate ones. The chapter provides guidance on how to develop personal strategies to challenge disrespectful behaviour, including bullying and recommends actions that can implemented to achieve culture change, with a summary of recommended actions given at the end of every section. The chapter provides vignettes, examples and case studies of how compassionate leaders have achieved culture change in the workplaces they are responsible for.

## 1.6    Conclusion

Exercises, vignettes and case studies are included throughout the book. Whether you are a student or a member of staff, to engage in the exercises will provide an opportunity for you to realise your strengths and areas for personal growth within your professional careers and personal lives.

> **Box 1.1 Exercise: Does Disrespectful Behaviour Occur Where You Work and Are You Confident to Challenge It?**
> Please reflect on your own workplace.
> Have you experienced being treated insensitively by another member of staff?
> Have you witnessed someone else being treated in a way that you perceive to be insensitive?
> If you answered yes to either or both questions, how did these experiences make you feel?
> Did you feel able to challenge the member of staff on behalf of yourself?
> Did you feel able to challenge the member of staff on behalf of the other person?

This exercise establishes whether you believe disrespectful behaviour occurs within your workplace and how confident you feel to challenge it. We will revisit this in the final chapter, Finding Resolution, to determine, after reading this book, whether your confidence has increased by undertaking the exercises, reading the vignettes, case studies and examples given by compassionate leaders for achieving positive cultures in maternity and neonatal services.

## References


Ball L, Curtis, P, Kirkham M (2002) Why do midwives leave? London, England: Royal College of Midwives

Begley C M (2002) 'Great fleas have little fleas': Irish student midwives' views of the hierarchy in midwifery Journal of Advanced Nursing 38 (3):310–317

Burleigh A, Wylam J, Millar B, Gillen P, Webster J, McEwen K, Gayle E, Hughes D, Lawrie A (2023) #Saynotobullyinginmidwifery. Available: www.midwifery.org.uk/news/support/saynotobullyinginmidwifery-report/ (accessed 26 Jan 2025)

Capper T S, Thorn M, Muurlink O T (2022). Workplace violence in the Australian and New Zealand midwifery workforce: A scoping review. Journal of Nursing Management, 30(6): 1831–1842. Available: https://doi.org/10.1111/jonm.13766 (Accessed 26 Feb 2025)

Capper T (2021) Workplace bullying: The midwifery student experience [Online]. CQ University Australia. Available: https://acquire.cqu.edu.au/articles/thesis/Workplace_bullying_The_midwifery_student_experience/14776482/1/files/28395063.pdf (accessed 14 August 2024)

Catling C, Reid F, Hunter B (2017) Australian midwives' experiences of their workplace culture. Women and Birth. 30(2):137–145 Available: https://doi.org/10.1016/j.wombi.2016.10.001 (Accessed 25 Feb 2025)

Catling C, Rossiter C (2020) Midwifery workplace culture in Australia: A national survey of midwives. Women and Birth 33: 464–472. Available: https://pubmed.ncbi.nlm.nih.gov/31676324/ (accessed 27 Jan 2025)

Care Quality Commission (2024). National Review of Maternity Service 2022 – 2024 available: https://www.cqc.org.uk/publications/maternity-services-2022-2024 (accessed 26 Jan 2025)

Coaching in Mind (2025) Available at https://coachesinmind.com/ (accessed 27 Feb 2025)

Commission for Healthcare Audit and Inspection (2006) Investigation into 10 Maternal Deaths, or Following Delivery at, North West London Hospitals NHS Trust between April 2002 and April 2005. London: England. Available: https://minhalexander.com/wp-content/uploads/2016/09/hcc-northwick-park-_tagged.pdf (accessed 26th Jan 2025)

Darzi A (2024). Independent Investigation of the National Health Service in England. Crown Copyright: England. Available: https://www.gov.uk/government/publications/independent-investigation-of-the-nhs-in-england (accessed 26 Jan 2025)

Feeley C, Stacey T (2024) Novel solutions to the midwifery retention crisis in England: an organisational case study of midwives' intentions to leave the profession and the role of retention midwives. Midwifery. Available: https://doi.org/10.1016/j.midw.2024.104152 (accessed 28 Jan 2025)

Francis R (2013) Report of the Mid Staffordshire NHS Foundation Trust public inquiry: executive summary [online] The Stationary Office. Available: https://assets.publishing.service.gov.uk/government/uploads/system/uploads/attachment_data/file/279124/0947.pdf (accessed 26 Jan 2025)

Gillen P Sinclair M, Kernohan WG (2008) The nature and manifestations of bullying in midwifery. Belfast: Ulster University. Available: https://pure.ulster.ac.uk/ws/portalfiles/portal/101327391/Gillen_2008_bullying.pdf (accessed 26 Jan 2025)

Gillen P, Sinclair M, Kernohan GW, Begley C (2009) 'Student midwives' experience of bullying'. Evidence-Based Midwifery, 7(2):46+. Available: https://link.gale.com/apps/doc/A204894578/HRCA?u=anon~4ec74bf6&sid=googleScholar&xid=08e2bf29 (accessed 27 Jan 2025)

Hadikin R, O'Driscoll M (2000). The bullying culture: cause, effect, harm reduction. Books for Midwives Press: Oxford, England

Independent Maternity Review (2022) Ockenden report – Final: Findings, conclusions, and essential actions from the independent review of maternity services at the Shrewsbury and Telford Hospital NHS Trust (HC 1219) Crown. Available: https://assets.publishing.service.gov.uk/government/uploads/system/uploads/attachment_data/file/1064302/Final-Ockenden-Report-web-accessible.pdf (accessed 30 August 2024)

Johnston J (2016) The lived experiences of student midwives subjected to inappropriate behaviour [Online]. University of Southampton. Available: https://eprints.soton.ac.uk/411282/1/Jane_Johnston_Thesis.pdf (accessed 27 Jan 2025)

Kirkup B (2022) Reading the signals, Maternity and Neonatal Services East Kent – the report of the independent investigation. London: His Majesty's Stationary Office Available: https://assets.publishing.service.gov.uk/media/634fb083e90e0731a5423408/reading-the-signals-maternity-and-neonatal-services-in-east-kent_the-report-of-the-independent-investigation_print-ready.pdf (accessed 27 Jan 2025)

Kirkup B (2015) The Report of the Morecambe Bay Investigation. Available at: http://data.parliament.uk/DepositedPapers/Files/DEP2015-0267/The_Report_of_the_Morecambe_Bay.pdf (accessed 27 Jan 2025)

Kitson-Reynolds, E. (2010). The Lived Experience of Newly Qualified Midwives. Thesis, University of Southampton

Kitson-Reynolds E (2020) The University of Southampton Midwifery Values Based Enquiry Journey. University of Southampton: Southampton

Maben J, Taylor C, Reynolds E, McCarthy I, Leamy M (2021) Realist evaluation of Schwartz Rounds for enhancing the delivery of compassionate healthcare: understanding how they work, for whom, and in what contexts. BMC Health Serv. Res.21 (709)

McNeil M, Kitson-Reynolds E (2024). Student midwives' experiences of clinical placement and the decision to enter the professional register. British Journal of Midwifery 32:14–20. Available: https://www.britishjournalofmidwifery.com/content/research/student-midwives-experiences-of-clinical-placement-and-the-decision-to-enter-the-professional-register/ (accessed 26 Jan 2025)

Mayra K, Catling C, Musa H, Hunter B, Baird K (2023) Compassion for midwives: The missing element in workplace culture for midwives globally. PLOS Glob Public Health 3(7): e0002034. https://doi.org/10.1371/journal.pgph.0002034

Mills and Reeve (2021) Mills & Reeve Achieve more. Together. New NHS patient safety strategy: The 'golden thread'. Available: https://www.mills-reeve.com/blogs/health-and-care/july-2019/new-nhs-patient-safety-strategy-the-golden-thread/ (accessed 28 Feb 2025)

NHS England (2018) News. Avoidable patient harm to be halved in key areas as a part of ambitious strategy. Available: https://www.england.nhs.uk/2018/12/avoidable-patient-harm-to-be-halved-in-key-areas-as-part-of-ambitious-strategy/ (Accessed 28 Feb 2025)

Nursing and Midwifery Council (2019) Standards for Pre-registration Midwifery Programmes. Nursing and Midwifery Council, London. Available: https://www.nmc.org.uk/globalassets/sitedocuments/standards/2024/standards-of-proficiency-for-midwives.pdf (Accessed 24 Feb 2025)

Oates J, Topping A, Watts K, (2020) 'The rollercoaster': A qualitative study of midwifery students' experiences affecting their mental wellbeing. Midwifery 88. https://doi.org/10.1016/j.midw.2020.102735

O'Brien M (2018a) Developing a Compassionate Workplace. Presentation presented at the Northern Maternity and Midwifery Festival, Manchester. 26 June 2018

O'Brien M (2018b) Respectful Relationships in Maternity Services. Presentation presented at the Northern Maternity and Midwifery Festival. Manchester. 26 June 2018

O'Brien M (2018c) Practical Steps to Developing a Respectful and Caring Workplace: Challenging Bullying Behaviours. Cardiff. 20 Sept 2018

Oxford English Dictionary (2025) Oxford University Press. Oxford Available at: https://www.oxfordlearnersdictionaries.com/definition/english/golden-thread?q=golden+thread  (Accessed 28 Feb 2025)

Ockenden D (2020) Ockenden Report. Emerging Findings and Recommendations from the Independent Review of Maternity Services at the Shrewsbury and Telford hospital NHS Trust. HMSO, London. Available: https://assets.publishing.service.gov.uk/media/5fd20f8be90e076637bb5a24/Independent_review_of_maternity_services_at_Shrewsbury_and_Telford_Hospital_NHS_Trust.pdf. (Accessed 26 Jan 2025)

Rogers H, Linay D (2025) Coaches in Mind. Available at: https://coachesinmind.com/ (Accessed 26 Feb 2025)

Royal College Midwives (1996) In place of fear: recognising and confronting the problem of bullying in midwifery RCM, London, England

Royal College Midwives (2016) Why midwives leave – revisited. RCM. London, England. Available: https://cdn.ps.emap.com/wp-content/uploads/sites/3/2016/10/Why-Midwives-Leave.pdf (Accessed 26 Jan 2025)

Smith J (2021) Nurturing Maternity Staff. How to tackle trauma, stress and burnout to create a positive working culture in the NHS. Pinter and Martin, UK

The Point of Care Foundation (2025) Schwartz Rounds. Available: http://www.pointofcarefoundation.org.uk/our-work/Schwartz-rounds/ (accessed 4 Feb 2025)

West MA, Bailey S (2022) What is Compassionate Leadership. The Kings Fund https://www.kingsfund.org.uk/insight-and-analysis/long-reads/what-is-compassionateleadership (Accessed 25 Feb 2025)

West MA (2021) Compassionate Leadership: Sustaining Wisdom, Humanity and Presence Health and Social Care. London: Swirling Leaf Press

West MA, Eckert R, Collins B, Chowla R (2017) Caring to change: how compassionate leadership can stimulate innovation in health care 2017. The Kings Fund Available: https://assets.kingsfund.org.uk/f/256914/x/0b76247d02/caring_to_change_2017.pdf. (Accessed 24 Feb 2025)

West MA, Chowla R (2017) Compassionate leadership for compassionate health care. In P Gilbert (ed.), Compassion: Concepts, Research and Applications. Routledge, London, pp. 237–257. Available: https://doi.org/10.4324/9781315564296 Accessed 26 Feb 2022

Wylam (2023) Why do Newly Qualified and Student Midwives Leave. In A Barrett, A Burleigh, P Gillen, D Hughes (Eds.) #saynotobullyinginmidwifery (pp 116–199). Available: www.midwifery.org.uk/news/support/saynotobullyinginmidwifery-report/ (accessed 26 Jan 2025)

# Where Are We Now?

**2**

Maggie O'Brien

## 2.1 Introduction

This chapter provides a background and context to the book through reviewing published research evidence and exploring maternity service reviews and investigations. It establishes that disrespectful behaviour, including bullying, has existed within maternity units for many years and examines how disrespectful cultures may impact women and birthing people and maternity staff. It explains how cultures develop and evolve, highlighting how those disrespectful behaviours and sometimes bullying and harassment flourish in negative cultures. The differences between disrespectful behaviour, bullying, harassment and discrimination are identified, as it is hoped that by acquiring a knowledge and understanding of the differences between these behaviours and their detrimental effects that anyone who has been, or is currently being or feeling targeted, will understand that they are not to blame; it is the permissive culture in which they are working that is usually responsible.

If we are to ensure that all women and birthing people, maternity and neonatal staff are respected and valued, it will be necessary to change the culture of some maternity and neonatal units. We must achieve this quickly before more staff leave and potentially more harm occurs to women, birthing people and neonates.

> … we have made clear our finding that women and their families have suffered additional harm as a result of the behaviours and attitudes of the health professionals who were responsible for their care. (Kirkup 2022, p. 69)

M. O'Brien (✉)
University of Southampton, Southampton, United Kingdom

Royal College of Midwives RCMF (Hons), London, United Kingdom
e-mail: Mahues935@gmail.com


M. O'Brien, E. Kitson-Reynolds (eds.), *Respectful Relationships in the Maternity Service*, https://doi.org/10.1007/978-3-032-04281-1_2

## 2.2    Evidence of Disrespectful Cultures in Maternity Services

Research evidence has been published demonstrating that midwives have been subjected to disrespectful behaviour over many years, both in the United Kingdom (UK) (Burleigh et al. 2023; Royal College Midwives [RCM] 1996, 2016; Gillen et al. 2008; Curtis et al. 2003, 2006a, b, c, d, e, f; Ball et al. 2002; Hadikin and O'Driscoll 2000) and internationally (Catling et al. 2017; Catling and Rossiter 2020; Capper et al. 2022; Mayra et al. 2023). The RCM undertook the first large-scale research consisting of a questionnaire survey of 1000 randomly selected midwives from across the UK. The response rate was 46% ($n = 462$), with 43% ($n = 147$) stating that they had been subjected to bullying (RCM 1996). Midwives also reported anxiety, irritability and depression, with as many as 55% contemplating leaving their jobs and the profession as a direct result of bullying. Concerned by these findings, the RCM commissioned further research, resulting in the publication *Why do Midwives Leave?* (Ball et al. 2002), followed by a series of articles discussing and raising awareness of the findings of the research (Curtis et al. 2003, 2006a, b, c, d, e, f). In addition to midwives, students are sometimes treated disrespectfully both in the UK (McNeil and Kitson-Reynolds 2024; Wylam 2023; Oates et al. 2020; Johnson 2016; Kitson-Reynolds et al. 2014; Kitson-Reynolds 2010) and internationally (Begley 1999a, b, 2002; Capper 2021). There is conclusive research evidence (Gillen et al. 2008, 2009) that bullying behaviour directed towards students occurs both in practice and within universities. The research undertaken by Gillen et al. (2008) consisted of a self-administered survey questionnaire, sent to 400 student midwives. The questionnaire was developed from a literature review and a concept analysis undertaken as part of a doctoral thesis (Gillen et al. 2004); 41% ($n = 164$) of student midwives responded; of these 50% ($n = 82$) had either experienced or witnessed bullying. Usually, the perpetrator was a midwife or the student's mentor with some university lecturers and personal tutors also identified as perpetrators. The research highlighted the permissive cultures that exist within some maternity units and universities that allow bullying behaviour to flourish. The research finding that university lecturers and personal tutors were sometimes perpetrators was a new finding at that time, with more research recommended on the issue (Gillen et al. 2008). The consequence of student midwives working in negative cultures both in the UK and internationally is that many leave their midwifery programmes. The NHS England (NHSE) undertook a survey in 2022 with the finding that 58.2% of student midwives had considered leaving (NHSE 2022). Additionally, some student midwives do not register as midwives on the point of qualification (McNeil and Kitson-Reynolds 2024; Wylam 2023; Capper 2021). The financial costs of this for the student and the university are significant and for the NHS, there is a considerable impact on the future workforce and its ability to be able to provide maternity care in the foreseeable future.

Following the publication of the Francis Report (2013) and the Kirkup Report (2015) (see Sect. 2.3), significant efforts to change non-compassionate and unkind maternity and neonatal cultures were made through publications, workshops, forums and by developing strategies and awareness courses. At this time, Byrom and Downe (2015) edited the book *Roar behind the silence. Why kindness, compassion and respect matter in maternity care*, reflecting their philosophical belief that kindness and compassion are fundamental to high-quality maternity care. This significant publication explored examples of compassionate maternity care and became popular on an international basis, triggering 'Roar' events both in the UK and in maternity units across the world. The different initiatives to improve maternity cultures were successful in some maternity units, with Baroness Cumberledge stating in the report, *Better Births: Improving Outcomes of Maternity Services in England*, that 'great strides had been made in transforming maternity services' (NHSE 2016, p. 3); however, the level of compassionate care shown to women and birthing people and to staff varied greatly between NHS Trusts.

Despite the strongly supported campaign to raise awareness of the need to improve the culture of some maternity units, evidence of the continuing lack of compassion was provided again in 2016 by the RCM. This was through an online survey entitled *Why Midwives Leave Revisited* (RCM 2016). Of the 2719 responses, 30.8% ($n = 836$) of responses were from midwives who had left midwifery in the last 2 years and 69.2% ($n = 1882$) of responses were from midwives who are intending to leave midwifery within the next 2 years. The two main reasons for midwives leaving or thinking of leaving were poor staffing levels and the inability to provide the quality of care that midwives wanted to give. Shockingly, 19% ($n = 157$) of midwives who had already left gave bullying from colleagues as one of their main reasons for leaving, with 11% ($n = 92$) giving bullying from a manager.

In 2017, the #Saynotobullyinginmidwifery private Facebook support group was created by Amanda Burleigh and Dany Griffiths as a support for midwives, student midwives and maternity support workers (MSWs) who had been badly affected because of being bullied in their workplace. The #Saynotobullyinginmidwifery grew quickly and now has 4200 followers including students, MSWs and midwives of all levels including Heads of Midwifery (HOM). Members obtain support and advice when sharing their anonymised and often heart-breaking accounts of having suffered bullying or are currently experiencing being bullied. Often, the midwives who describe their experiences have left or decided to leave the midwifery profession altogether and many of the students who posted on the page have discontinued their training programmes. The Facebook page contains many examples of horizontal violence described by Leap (1997) as:

> … a scapegoating, backstabbing and negative criticism. The failure to respect privacy or keep confidences, non-verbal innuendo, undermining, lack of openness, unwillingness to help out and lack of support. (Leap 1997, p. 689)

In November 2023, the #Saynotobullyinginmidwifery group published a report/book (Burleigh et al. 2023). A team of authors from the Facebook group (led by Amanda) worked together to gather and collate accounts from members of the group. The report/book was published with the support of the Association of Radical Midwives (ARMS), the Independent Midwifery and Birth Education Trust (TIMBET) and others. The report/book consists of harrowing accounts of experiences of members of the Facebook group and is a powerful record of bullying, disrespectful behaviour and horizontal violence that currently exist in some maternity and neonatal units. The report was sent to significant Members of Parliament, HOMs, Directors of Midwifery (DOM), Universities, the Nursing and Midwifery Council (NMC), Chief Midwifery Officer and the RCM in an effort to raise awareness of the current serious situation. With the exception of a Member of Parliament who raised questions in the House of Lords, and a response from the Scottish government, there was no response from those mentioned above (Burleigh et al. 2023).

## 2.3 Maternity Unit Reviews in England

The disrespectful cultures that do not treat women and birthing people with kindness and lack of compassion is often reflected in the quality of maternity and neonatal care provided to women, birthing people and their families; this is evident from the reviews of maternity services over the last 20 years. There have been a series of reviews into failing maternity services since 2006. The first was at North West London Hospitals NHS Trust, which became the subject of two investigations by the Healthcare Commission (HCC) as a result of 10 maternal deaths occurring between April 2002 and April 2005 (Commission for Healthcare Audit and Inspection 2006). The HCC highlighted the link between negative cultures and patient safety, stating in one of its conclusions:

> Despite the good intentions of staff who were working in very difficult circumstances, their practice and ultimately the care they provided were compromised by the environment and the culture in which they were working. It was an environment that allowed the quality of care to fall below proper professional standards and poor working practices to flourish. (Commission for Healthcare Audit and Inspection 2006, p. 7)

As a result of the findings of the two investigations, the HCC called upon the Health Secretary to put the NHS Trust under special measures; this involved bringing in an outside team of experts to review the NHS Trust's maternity services to ensure patient safety. Additionally, quality standards across all NHS Trust's providing maternity services were required to be monitored by the HCC, with regular inspections carried out; these inspections, under different formats, were still undertaken in 2024, by the Care Quality Commission (CQC) (2024).

Concerns regarding quality of care across all NHS services were raised again in 2013 following a public enquiry, by Robert Francis QC, into serious failings at Mid Staffordshire NHS Foundation Trust (Francis 2013). Although not directly mentioning midwives, this reports states in its conclusion that a fundamental culture change was needed across the organisation. Following the Francis inquiry, concerns were raised about maternity services at University Hospitals of Morecambe Bay NHS Foundation Trust going back as far as 2004. Consequently, an independent investigation into the management, delivery and outcomes of care provided by the maternity and neonatal services at the University Hospitals of Morecambe Bay NHS Foundation Trust from January 2004 to June 2013 was undertaken. This investigation found 20 instances of significant failures that may have led to the deaths of three mothers and 16 babies. Both the Francis and Kirkup reports (Francis 2013; Kirkup 2015) raised similar concerns, with the Kirkup report recommending a national review of the provision of maternity care. This review, undertaken by Baroness Cumberledge, resulted in the publication of *Better Births: Improving outcomes of maternity services in England* (NHSE 2016). 'Better Births' (NHSE 2016) highlighted differences across England in the number of NHS Trusts providing compassionate and kind care (see Sect. 2.2). The quote from the report below aptly describes the situation across England at the time, together with the impact of insensitive language and dismissive remarks.

> When a baby dies, nothing can take away the pain for the families, but we heard many accounts of kind, compassionate care that made the experience better and helped parents to create positive memories. On the other hand, we heard too from families who said they were treated with a lack of care and kindness. Insensitive language and dismissive remarks lodged in parents' minds, causing hurt and polluting memories of the often very short time they had with their baby. (NHSE 2016, p. 4)

Then, in 2017, Jeremy Hunt, the former Secretary of Health for Health and Social Care, instructed NHS Improvement to commission a review assessing the quality of investigations relating to newborn, infant and maternal harm at Shrewsbury and Telford NHS Trust. In all, 1862 maternity cases were reviewed by Donna Ockendon, making it the largest clinical review in the history of the NHS (Independent Maternity Review 2022). The Independent Maternity Review (2022) identified the following themes as needing addressing:

1. Enhanced safety
2. Listening to women and their families
3. Staff training and working together
4. Managing complex pregnancy
5. Risk assessment throughout pregnancy
6. Monitoring foetal well-being

**Informed Consent** Following the publication of the Independent Maternity Review (2022), concerns were raised about the numbers of baby deaths that had occurred at East Kent Hospitals University NHS Foundation Trust. Nadine Dorries, MP, then Minister for Patient Safety, commissioned another independent inquiry, this time led by Bill Kirkup; 202 cases were examined, resulting in the publication of the report *Reading the signals, Maternity and Neonatal Services East Kent—the report of the independent investigation* (Kirkup 2022). The findings of this report are shocking, echoing the findings of previous reports and stating that a lack of kindness and compassion causes harm to women and birthing people.

> Nor was the harm restricted to physical damage. Chapter 3 sets out the equally disturbing effects of the repeated lack of kindness and compassion on the wider experience of families, both as care was given and later in the aftermath of injuries and deaths. (Kirkup 2022, p. 2)

The most recent CQC report, *National Review of Maternity Services Report 2022–2024* (CQC 2024), made findings from 131 maternity inspections; as with the findings of the NHS England (2016) 'Better Births' report, the CQC 'identified pockets of excellent practice', with variable ratings across England; 4% rated outstanding, 48% rated good, 36% rated requires improvement and 12% rated inadequate.

## 2.4    The Importance of Achieving Kindness and Compassion for Women and Birthing People

The Independent Maternity Review (2022) acknowledges the impact that some maternity staff have made with their kindness and compassion:

> There are some examples of midwives and doctors who have made a huge difference to the women and families due to the care they provided and kindness they showed. (Independent Maternity Review 2022, p. 11)

It then gives many examples of where kindness and compassion are lacking (Independent Maternity Review 2022, pp. 116–117). Chapter 3 of the Kirkup Report (Kirkup 2022) is entitled *The Wider Experience of the Families* with findings and examples grouped into six themes identified below (Kirkup 2022, p. 38):

1. Not being listened to or consulted with
2. Encountering a lack of kindness and compassion
3. Being conscious of unprofessional conduct or poor working relationships compromising their care
4. Feeling excluded during and immediately after a serious event
5. Feeling ignored, marginalised or disparaged after a serious event
6. Being forced to live with an incomplete or inaccurate narrative

The findings identified within theme two above 'Encountering a lack of kindness and compassion' are grouped into the following categories, with examples given within the report to illustrate the lack of kindness and compassion:

1. Showing a basic lack of kindness, care and understanding to women and their families
2. Making unkind or insensitive comments to women and their partners
3. Showing an indifference to women's pain
4. Failing to ensure or preserve women's dignity or provide for their basic needs
5. Placing women with other mothers and their newborn babies following the loss of their own baby or after a serious event
6. Putting pressure on families to consent to a post-mortem examination

The examples of behaviours and actions given within the report (Kirkup 2022, pp. 47–51) are shocking, difficult to read and, undoubtably, have a lasting detrimental impact upon women and birthing people and their families. During the writing of this book, opinions of how lack of kindness and compassion from maternity staff impacts women and birthing people were sought from an ex-chair of a Maternity Voices group. They felt strongly about the importance of kindness and compassion, describing experiences they and other members of their Maternity Voices group had raised. The examples of lack of kindness and compassion given include the following:

1. Midwives having heated discussions about the woman or birthing person in front of them with everyone on the ward able to hear
2. Partners of women and birthing people being ignored and left to struggle in theatre changing rooms and in theatre itself
3. Black and Asian women and birthing people being treated differently; a local survey was undertaken with differences in care highlighted, including preconceived ideas of the lifestyle of Black and Asian women; for example, being asked multiple times about their use of contraception because 'Black women have lots of babies'
4. Asking all Black and Asian women and birthing people if they are required to pay for NHS care, but not asking White women and birthing people at all
5. No consideration of ethnicity, for example, the type of food offered, with no knowledge and understanding of religious beliefs and customs

**Box 2.1 Vignette: Impact of Lack of Kindness and Compassion on Women and Birthing People**

Valerie had given birth the day before to her first baby, Noah, and was feeling exhausted, apprehensive and anxious about whether she would be able to breastfeed successfully. She had developed a good relationship with the midwife who had supported her to breastfeed and was beginning to develop some confidence that Noah was fixing well on the nipple. It was usual practice on the postnatal ward, that a handover between the midwife who had responsibility for Valerie's care and the midwife arriving on duty and assuming responsibility took place at lunch time every day. The time arrived for the handover, Helen, the early-shift midwife, and Tina, the late-shift midwife, met at the end of Valerie's bed to start the handover. Valerie was breastfeeding Noah at the time of the handover and Helen had reassured her that he had fixed well on the nipple. Tina, however, had a different opinion and started to say in a loud voice with a harsh tone, that if Noah continued feeding as he was, Valerie would get sore nipples and suggested he have 'top-ups' of formula milk 'until Valerie's milk came in' and to 'give her nipples a rest'.

(continued)

**Box 2.1** (continued)

Helen strongly disagreed and the two midwives began to have a very heated discussion in front of Valerie and other women and birthing people in the four-bedded bay. Valerie began to inwardly feel very anxious and embarrassed, but did not feel confident to say anything. Tina seemed so sure that Valerie would get sore nipples because of excessive sucking and poor attachment that she started to question Helen's advice and think that she should phone her partner to ensure that she had some sterilised bottles and formula milk for when she arrived home. Tina took over Valerie's care and gave her different advice with regard to breastfeeding from what Helen had given, informing Valerie that Helen was a newly qualified midwife who had no experience of breastfeeding, with no children of her own. Tina continued to explain that she, on the other hand, had been qualified 20 years, had three children of her own and had to stop breastfeeding each time because of sore nipples. Tina was very abrupt to Valerie and did not speak well about her colleague.

As a result of Tina's behaviour, Valerie lost confidence in the advice Helen gave and, in her ability, to breastfeed; consequently, Noah was fully bottle-fed when Valerie was discharged home the following day.

## 2.5 The Importance of Achieving Inclusion

The latest data, provided by the 2020–2022 Mothers and Babies Reducing Risk through Audits, and Confidential Enquires across the UK (MBRRACE-UK) report (Felker et al. 2024), demonstrate that poor outcomes are higher for women and pregnant people and babies from Black and Asian ethnic groups. Maternal mortality is three times higher for Black women and two times higher for Asian women, than for a White woman (Felker et al. 2024).

> according to MBRRACE-UK data published in January 2024, Black women are still 2.8 times more likely to die during or up to 6 weeks after pregnancy compared with women in White ethnic groups. The data also showed that Asian women are 1.7 more times likely to die during the same period. Concerningly, we also found some trusts where both staff and people who were using the service experienced discrimination because of their ethnic background, or issues associated with having English as a second language or not their preferred language. (CQC 2024, p. 4)

In light of the poor outcomes for Black and Asian women and recent reports highlighting racism within the NHS (Darzi 2024) and maternity services (CQC 2024; Kirkup 2022), equity, diversity, inclusion and belonging (EDIB) have to be at the centre of decisions we make to ensure that maternity and neonatal services for all women and pregnant and birthing people and workplaces for all staff are truly inclusive and compassionate. This will involve changing our culture, including the language we use, the way we behave and the messages we communicate. A culture that values EDIB is more likely to be empathetic and compassionate and provide safe care because staff are more likely to feel psychologically safe (West 2021;

Smith 2021). Within an inclusive culture, everyone recognises that some people, due to their background, experiences or identity, are more likely to face challenges in everyday living, including exclusion, feeling unwelcome, devalued and being treated differently or unfairly compared to others. This in turn means that they are more vulnerable, resulting in having to face specific barriers to achieving the same health outcomes as everyone else. A diverse culture values and celebrates our differences, whatever they may be, whilst an inclusive and belonging culture is where equity and diversity meet to ensure that the actions we take and the cultures we create ensure everyone, whatever their background, feels comfortable and *confident to be the person they are*, welcomed, respected and valued. Inclusion is identified as 'a golden thread of change in this book' (OED 2025) (see Sect. 1.5), a quote from Jan Smith encapsulating everything that could be possible if inclusion is achieved, emphasising the link between inclusion and psychological safety:

> We have an opportunity in the UK to make genuine changes to ensure staff in maternity services are not just diverse, but also that the workspaces they occupy are inclusive. This means that it is psychologically and physically safe for *all* staff, irrespective of their race, gender, sexual or religious orientation, culture, disabilities, learning disabilities, neurodiversity and mental and physical challenges to be the person they are and values. (Smith 2021, p. 28)

The final chapter of this book looks at *how* inclusion can be achieved, and the importance of continuing to move forward in making it possible for everyone cannot be over emphasised, particularly as recent world events have put some of the hard-won achievements made over the last 20 years at risk.

## 2.6  The Importance of the Model of Care in Achieving Midwives' Well-Being

The model of midwifery care that a midwife works within is crucial to their well-being (Maben et al. 2023) (see Sect. 3.3.2) and often determines whether midwives and student midwives remain in midwifery (Curtis et al. 2006f; Feeley and Stacey 2024). The model of care is identified as 'a golden thread of change' (OED 2025) (see Sect. 1.5) because

> when there is an imbalance between what the perception of what the role *should* be and the reality, risking moral compromise, distress and/or injury when midwives are unable to provide the care birthing women and people deserve. (Feeley and Stacey 2024, p. 2)

Midwives have existed and been 'with women' throughout history (Verluysen 1980) and midwifery care would have been provided as individualised care for all women and birthing people, until the implementation of the NHS on 5 July 1948. This instigated the reorganisation of maternity care to come under the management of regional hospital boards, resulting in midwifery care becoming divided between hospital midwives and community midwives (O'Brien 2021, pp. 18–19). There ensued a gradual move of home birth to hospital birth and a medicalisation of care, for all women and birthing people, no matter whether they had complications or not, under the belief that hospital birth was safer than home birth for everyone (Tew 1989; Donnison 1988). Then, in 1990–1991, growing pressure from the National Childbirth Trust (NCT), Association of Improvement in Maternity Services (AIMS) and midwives resulted in the publication of the *Changing Childbirth Report* (DH 1993), which, if successfully implemented within the allotted 5-year time frame, would have radically transformed maternity services to give women more choice, continuity and control. The recommendations of the *Changing Childbirth Report* (DH 1993) were embraced by many midwives who were keen to change the fragmented model of maternity care, put women at the centre of care and reduce medicalisation. However, some midwives believed that the change to their lives was too great, with an on-call commitment causing stress and burn-out (Turner 2021; Sandall 1997). Many pilot schemes were commenced that provided evidence to support that quality of care, clinical outcomes and maternal satisfaction improve when women receive continuity of care (Sandall 2017; Sandall et al. 2016; Page 2003). However, the introduction of austerity, no resources given for implementation, together with the division within the maternity workforce meant that the aspiration of achieving choice, continuity and control for all women and birthing people was not achievable for all (O'Brien 2021).

The process of making significant recommendations to maternity units to improve the quality of care with no extra resource to support implementation has been repeated more recently, in that, one of the recommendations of *Better Births: Improving Outcomes of Maternity Services in England* (NHSE 2016) was that all women and birthing people should receive continuity of care. This recommendation was reinforced by the 2019 NHS Plan (NHS 2019). A programme of change was planned with DH targets set for NHS Trust maternity services to implement continuity of care, with pilot schemes again commenced with some senior midwives reorganising maternity services to implement the recommendation. However, once again, there was a strong difference of opinion within the midwifery workforce and no resources were provided to assist with the implementation. Then, in 2022, the Ockenden Report (Independent Maternity Review 2022, p. 179) recommended that due to a lack of staff and resources and for the safety of women and birthing people, the roll out of continuity of care should be 'reviewed and suspended if necessary', resulting in the closure of many of the schemes, through no fault of those who had worked hard to plan and implement them. Of course, the safety of the service must come first, but the effect of starting continuity of care projects that improve maternal satisfaction and clinical outcomes, then for them to be disbanded due to lack of funding and staffing has had a detrimental effect on morale and resulted in some midwives practising in ways they are ideologically misaligned to. It is important to emphasise that several successful continuity schemes are still running across the UK, with midwives providing continuity for many women and birthing people. The requirement for midwives to promote continuity is currently still explicit within Domain 2 of the NMC Standards of Proficiency for Midwives (NMC 2019, p. 16).

The division within the midwifery workforce is explained by Feeley (2023) who discusses research undertaken by Hunter (2004) to explore midwives accounts of 'emotional labour' when caring for women and birthing people:

> … established that two coexisting and conflicting ideologies of midwifery existed; 'with-women' and 'with institution'. Those aligned with occupational ideology were most associated with hospital-based midwifery driven by the needs of the institution, wherein standardised care, risk reduction, efficiency and effectiveness were valued most. Conversely, those aligned with a woman-centred ideology, associated with community-based midwifery driven by the needs of birthing women or people, wherein individualised care and physiological birth were valued. (Feeley 2023, p. 23)

The coexistence of two conflicting ideologies explains midwives' strong reactions to being asked to change the way in which they practise, either from fragmented hospital-based care to community-based care and vice versa. The model of care in which a midwife practises can impact their well-being (see Sect. 3.3.1). Smith (2021) cites Hunter et al. (2019) in discussing the mental health and well-being of midwives:

> In the case of midwives, evidence has suggested that younger, recently qualified midwives are at risk of personal burnout and experiencing heightened symptoms of anxiety and depression, one potential explanation for this is there is a mismatch between newly qualified midwives' ideals of midwifery work and the reality of working in maternity care. (Smith 2021, p. 2)

The midwifery model of care can be a source of conflict because 'some practitioners embrace one paradigm but tend to practice according to the other due to the cultural norms in their practice settings. This may create dissonance' (Hunter 2004, p. 264). Hunter (2005) ascertains that 'it would seem that tackling a bullying culture will require attention to the fundamental ideological underpinnings of practice addressing any paradoxes that exist'.

When considering Hunter's (2004, 2005, 2010) findings, to achieve positive culture change, it is important that opportunities exist for midwives to practise in ways they are fundamentally aligned to; this is explored further in the final chapter, where we look finding resolution.

When reflecting on your own practice, are you aware if your ideology tends towards 'standardised care, risk reduction, efficiency and effectiveness' or 'the needs of birthing women or people and individualised care'? You may value each philosophy equally or one more than the other. Neither philosophy is 'right' or 'wrong'; maternity services need midwives of both philosophies to provide care to all women and birthing people whose maternity care will range from requiring complex care, due to medical or obstetric complications, to choosing to have a home birth; the key to avoiding conflict is for maternity service managers and individual members of staff to understand and accept that neither philosophy is more 'important' than the other and for opportunities to exist in ways midwives are ideologically aligned to.

## 2.7 Achieving Positive Cultures: Essential to Improving Care for Women and Birthing People and Staff Well-Being

> Efforts to bring about fundamental change in maternity care must acknowledge and develop strategies to deal with the culture of midwifery. (Kirkham 1999, p. 738)

Earlier research publications focused on raising awareness of bullying within midwifery (see Sect. 2.1) and its devastating impact (Hadikin and O'Driscoll 2000; Begley 1999a, b, 2002; RCM 1996). It then became evident that disrespectful behaviour and bullying were part of wider cultural issues, initially recognised by Kirkham (1999) and Curtis et al. (2006a) who published *Bullying and Horizontal Violence: Cultural or Individual Phenomena?* which discussed the finding that HOMs recognised bullying as a symptom of negative cultures. The more recent investigations and reviews of maternity services (Kirkup 2015, 2022; Independent Maternity Review 2022; CQC 2024) focus on cultural change as essential to improving maternity and neonatal services culture, safety and the quality of maternity and neonatal care.

### 2.7.1 How Cultures Develop

Cultures either develop or evolve as respectful and inclusive, where staff want to come to work or as intimidating and unkind where staff are scared to work, unless they are part of the 'power' dynamic that is central to the development of the culture. Disrespectful and bullying behaviours are common in negative, permissive cultures, often going unchallenged, due to fear of becoming the next victim and a desire to *fit in*. 'The need for belonging reflects our desire to feel and be connected to others' (West 2021). The beginnings of any culture may start with the introduction of one or two people who begin to develop a power base. It will depend on the values and ethos of these people whether the culture develops as a negative or a positive one. 'Power in itself is not an issue; it's how we use it that is dangerous to ourselves and others' (Smith 2021, p. 106).

Sometimes people are required to act in a certain way because of the culture, values and management of the wider organisation, with particular people appointed because they fit in with the ethos of the unit or department and are required to act in a 'controlling' way. Staff working in the unit/department start to 'role-model' the behaviour of the staff member holding the power, culminating in an expanding culture of fear and intimidation; 'In an effort to "fit in" and draw attention to oneself, it is desirable to become one of the gang' (Hadikin and O'Driscoll 2000, p. 55). Hunter (2005, p. 264) cites Kirkham (1999) in explaining how aggressive behaviour is displayed towards midwives whose 'views are considered to deviate from cultural norms', who, because of this aggressive behaviour, then 'reject their own principles and identity'. The culture slowly grows, like the ripples created when a stone is thrown into a pond, as more staff and sadly students begin to change their behaviour, the way in which they practise and even their values to 'fit in' to the culture.

Horizontal violence (Leap 1997, p. 689) (see Sect. 2.2) is often rife when this power dynamic is evident; the longer the culture is in place and allowed to flourish, the more embedded it becomes. Any attempts at innovation and change are believed to be unnecessary, everything 'is kept the same' because change is not in the interests of the staff holding the power. Where the culture is kind, compassionate and inclusive, staff are encouraged to be innovative and inspirational, resulting in dynamic care for women and birthing people.

For staff to survive practising within a negative culture, they either must change their behaviour to 'fit in' and become 'part of the gang' or leave the unit or department. To work differently and challenge embedded practices and behaviour can be detrimental to a staff member's mental health and well-being. To be on the 'outside of the culture' can cause long-term physiological and psychological harm to staff (Manufacturing Science Finance [MSF] Trade Union 1995; RCM 1996; Burleigh et al. 2023) and the trauma caused in these circumstances should not be underestimated. This, of course, applies to all staff, including doctors and MSWs, depending on who holds the power in a particular area.

> Going to work became harder and harder. I would have to make a choice each shift—a choice between being accepted by my colleagues or providing good midwifery care. (Smith 2021, p. 63)

Often, newly qualified midwives start their midwifery careers with a passion to provide excellent, women-centred care, but cannot maintain their enthusiasm within a negative culture. They will start out motivated and keen, but as their philosophy of 'how it should be' for women and birthing people is challenged by some of their colleagues, maternity unit polices and guidelines and sometimes managers, they can become disillusioned and lose their motivation. If, on the other hand, the culture is supportive, compassionate and innovative, these midwives will experience the joy of midwifery (Crowther 2020; McAra-Couper et al. 2014) be encouraged to develop their midwifery expertise and continue to practise and develop as a midwife.

Tall poppy syndrome originated in Australia and describes an innovative, curious, inspirational member of staff, advocating for change (a tall poppy) who, because of their success and growth, is the target of jealousy and grudging remarks; this person is likened to a tall poppy because *tall poppies are the first to be cut down*. Where tall poppy syndrome exists, there is a lack of innovation and change, for example, implementation of evidence-based practice, due to others being frightened to *shine* in fear of being *cut down*. The result is no one strives to achieve or even believe that change is possible. The long-term effect is midwives stop supporting each other to develop and progress and are cut down through constant criticism, ostracism and horizontal violence. This makes changes to culture and practice very difficult to implement, resulting in *everything staying the same;* tall poppy syndrome is common in negative, disrespectful cultures (Elliott 2004).

**Box 2.2 Vignette: The Effect of Tall Poppy Syndrome on Advocacy for Women and Birthing People**

Vanessa, a midwife who qualified 2 years ago, worked as a community midwife providing antenatal and postnatal care to a defined group of women and birthing people. Vanessa believed passionately in informed choice for women and birthing people and had supported and attended three home births for women and birthing people who had no obstetric or medical complications.

Mary is 9 weeks pregnant, has had two uncomplicated pregnancies and births and has decided to have a water birth. She attended her booking appointment with Vanessa where they discussed available research evidence regarding labouring and birthing in water; Vanessa explained to Mary that because her two previous pregnancies and labours progressed well with no complications and all was well with this pregnancy that she supported her choice. The NHS Trust policy, at that time, was that women and birthing people whose choice was to give birth in water were required to go into the birthing suite at the local maternity unit; Vanessa informed Mary of this policy who then asked Vanessa if she would be the midwife at the birth. Vanessa agreed to this, provided the pregnancy continued to progress well, with no complications.

Mary's pregnancy did progress well, Vanessa informed the maternity unit that Mary would be requiring the pool and her line manager that Mary had asked her to be the midwife at the birth. Mary went into labour naturally at 39 weeks. Mary and her partner made their way to the birthing suite and Vanessa met her there. On arrival, Mary was having strong contractions every 3 min and was keen to get into the pool to use water for pain relief. A midwife greeted them in the reception area, walked up to Mary and said, 'Oh you are the woman that wants a waterbirth', rolling her eyes at Vanessa. Although good warning had been given of their arrival, the midwife then said, 'you will need to wait in the reception area whilst we get the pool room ready' and left Vanessa, Mary and her partner in the reception area. They waited 10 min by which time Mary was contracting strongly every 2 min and her membranes had ruptured.

Vanessa went to see if the room was ready, encountering the midwife who had met them together with two midwives sitting at the midwives' station, talking amongst themselves. Vanessa asked if the room was ready and was told, 'in about 15 min' as the MSW was cleaning it. All three midwives then started asking Vanessa if she knew that water births were 'unsafe' and asking why she had supported Mary to have one. The verbal attack was loud, and Vanessa felt her confidence draining away, suddenly feeling very nervous. Vanessa replied that her manager had told her that she would receive support from the midwives on duty. The midwives laughed saying, 'they were not experienced in waterbirths' and carried on their own conversations. Vanessa helped the MSW to finish cleaning the room and began to run the water into

(continued)

> **Box 2.2** (continued)
>
> the pool. She returned to the reception area and took Mary and her partner to the pool room, Mary, by this time, was wanting to push. They made it to the room but not the pool and a baby boy was born on the bed in the room. He cried at birth, had skin to skin with Mary and breast feeding was initiated within 5 min. Mary had no complications, but was disappointed because she did not have the water birth she had dreamed of.

This case study uses pseudonyms, but is a true account of a situation that occurred in a maternity unit about 15 years ago. The midwife coordinators who worked on the birthing suite did not feel confident to assist women and birthing people to give birth in water, so they made assisting a woman or birthing person to give birth in water as difficult as possible for midwives through criticism and ostracism. This resulted in only three waterbirths in the NHS Trust that year. Vanessa was traumatised by the events that had occurred, which resulted in changing her practice to stop supporting women and birthing people who requested a waterbirth; she also developed a fear of working on the birthing unit. Vanessa eventually left the NHS Trust and is now practising in a unit that supports women and birthing people's informed choice. The implication for women and birthing people living in the area the NHS Trust provides maternity care for is that they have no choice regarding labouring and birthing in water in the maternity unit, even though the midwifery managers profess to support it.

## 2.7.2 Is It Disrespectful or Bullying Behaviour?

It is important to be able to recognise the difference between disrespectful and bullying behaviour; once understood, it is easier to identify if someone is bullying you, and to support a member of staff to identify bullying behaviour. It is important for a manager undertaking an investigation into an allegation of bullying from a member of staff, to be able to determine whether bullying did occur. Almost everyone will have 'bad days' where they go to work stressed and/or upset due to either a personal or work issue; the work issues that cause staff to become stressed are explored further (see Chap. 3). The disrespectful behaviour displayed could be one or more of the examples given below; if there is a compassionate culture within the workplace and the behaviour displayed is considered unacceptable, another member of staff will feel safe to 'step in' and 'defuse' the situation. If something either personally or work related had happened to cause the staff member to behave disrespectfully, it is important to support them. In compassionate cultures, when the staff member becomes aware of how they have behaved, they usually apologise to anyone impacted by their behaviour (O'Brien 2018b).

### 2.7.3 What Is Disrespectful Behaviour?

Examples of disrespectful behaviour were first defined by the MSF trade union (MSF 1995) and have evolved over years with experience gained of managing staff behaviour; the examples of disrespectful behaviour remain relevant today:

*Open aggression*, threats, shouting abuse and/or obscenities
*Constant humiliation* or ridicule, often in front of others
*Deliberately withholding information*, which the person requires to do their job effectively
*Refusing reasonable requests for leave*, training, etc. or blocking a persons' promotion
*Ostracising and marginalising*
*Setting impossible objectives* or constantly changing the work remit without telling the person, and then criticising them
*Excessive supervision* and being excessively critical about minor things
*Constantly taking credit for the other person's work*, but never taking the blame when things go wrong
*Spreading malicious rumours* and making personal remarks

There are, of course, many different examples of disrespectful behaviour, and there are also differences between friendly chat, unkind chatter and malicious talk:

- *Friendly chat*—here is no intention to cause offense and no one is upset.
- *Unkind gossip*—'crosses the line' with no intent to hurt; the perpetrator will often apologise.
- *Malicious talk*—done with the intention to humiliate a person, often in front of others.

### 2.7.4 Definition of Bullying Behaviour

Bullying behaviour can be one or many of the examples of disrespectful behaviour described above, but it usually targets one person; it can either happen in front of other members of staff and/or women and birthing people or it can be insidious and only happen where no one else is aware of what is happening. The RCM gave one of the first definitions of bullying in midwifery in their publication *In place of fear: recognising and confronting the problem of bullying in midwifery* (RCM 1996). This was adapted from the MSF trade union definition:

> Persistent, offensive, abusive, intimidating, malicious or insulting behaviour, abuse of power or unfair penal sanctions, which makes the recipient feel upset, threatened, humiliated or vulnerable, which undermines their self-confidence and which may cause them to suffer stress. (MSF 1995, p. 6)

Although this definition is accurate, it was still difficult to prove or disprove whether bullying had occurred. Then, in 2004, Gillen et al. (2004) recognised the need for a research-based definition, stating in their concept analysis of bullying in midwifery that 'uncertainty remains as to an agreed definition of bullying, which is a prerequisite for any agreed action. This lack of clarity leads to uncertainty in research, policy and practice' (Gillen et al. 2004, p. 46). The concept analysis defined four attributes that made it possible to determine whether, or not, bullying had occurred. Gillen et al. (2004) concluded in their concept analysis that bullying was complex and crossed personal and professional boundaries; it identified four defining attributes of bullying behaviour that must be present if bullying is said to have occurred:

1. The repeated nature of the behaviour.
2. Negative effect of the behaviour on the victim.
3. The victim finds it difficult to defend themselves (power imbalance).
4. Intent of the bully.

To validate the findings of the concept analysis, focus groups consisting of midwives, student midwives, midwife managers, academic midwives and union representatives were used as an inductive confirmatory process of the four defining attributes (Gillen et al. 2008). The four defining attributes were validated in the context of midwifery and a new definition of bullying in midwifery was developed as a result of the research findings:

> Bullying in midwifery is the *often intentional, repeated*, persistent, offensive, abusive. intimidating, malicious or insulting behaviour, abuse of power or unfair penal sanctions *against which the victim finds it difficult to defend themselves*. It *has a negative effect on the recipient* which makes the feel upset, threatened, humiliated or vulnerable; undermines their self-confidence and which may cause them to suffer stress. (Gillen et al. 2008, p. 16)

**The Repeated Nature of the Behaviour**  There are differing opinions over whether to be considered bullying, behaviour has to be repeated (Hadikin and O'Driscoll 2000). Gillen et al.'s (2004) research found that behaviour has to be repeated for it to be defined as bullying behaviour. This view took account of the opinions of other authors (RCM 1996; RCN 1996) that it is the repeated nature of the behaviour that makes it so harmful to the victim, including causing anxiety by making them continually wanting to please the perpetrator. Remember that bullying comes in many forms, both overt and insidious, all of which must be taken into account when undertaking an investigation to determine if bullying has occurred.

**Negative Effect of the Behaviour**  The student midwives who participated in the forums described harmful effects, which included those seriously impacting their physical and mental health, with a devastating revelation from one student who had contemplated taking their own life (Gillen et al. 2008).

**Difficulty in Defending Self**  Power imbalance affects the victim's ability to defend themselves with bullies being dependent on this to perpetuate the cycle. The cycle is based on the perpetrator drawing strength from harming the victim enabling them to increase the attacks on the victim by the bully. 'There was a clear power imbalance between the student midwives and qualified staff in both clinical practice and university settings' (Gillen et al. 2008, p. 15).

**Intent of the Bully**  This can be difficult to measure, but the majority of staff who participated in the forums who had been bullied believed that the perpetrator intended to bully them.

---

**Box 2.3 Vignette: Returning from Maternity Leave**

The following vignette is a true description of Susan's (pseudonym) first shift on her return to work following maternity leave in 1988.

Susan arrived at the local maternity unit for a night shift as a midwife, her first since the birth of her son 9 months previously, at the same maternity unit. Susan had just left her 8-month-old son, for the first time, so was feeling a little emotional, and was slightly nervous as she had been away from clinical practice for 9 months but was looking forward to meeting up with her colleagues again and resuming her practice as a midwife. On arrival, she was allocated to work on the birthing unit, so went straight to the midwife's station for the hand over from the evening shift midwives. The birthing unit coordinator did not say anything to welcome Susan, although the other two midwives on the night shift were pleased to see her, one was a friend who had been in the same cohort as Susan when they were student midwives.

There were three women in labour, two were in early labour and one was about to have a forceps birth. The other two midwives were allocated the women in early labour and Susan was allocated the woman who was about to have a forceps birth. Susan asked the birthing unit coordinator if she could be reallocated to one of the other women explaining that her own recent birth had been a difficult forceps birth, which she was having problems coming to terms with and she would find it difficult to go straight to assist at a forceps birth. The coordinator replied that she would have to do that at some point and why not now? The other two midwives on shift heard this conversation but did not say anything.

Susan went to the delivery room where the late-shift midwife and doctor were preparing the woman for a forceps birth due to a delayed second stage. Susan froze and just stood there with the memories of her own birth washing over her. The late-shift midwife, unaware of this, thanked her for taking over and left the room. Thankfully, Susan's professionalism took over, she was able to support the woman and assist the doctor and all was well with the mother and baby. After the baby and placenta were born, Susan realised that she was shaking, and tears were rolling down her face. She went outside of the room to the midwife's station where the labour ward midwife was chatting with one of midwives, nobody said anything.

**Box 2.4 Exercise Defining Bullying Behaviour**

After reading the above vignette and by applying the defining attributes described above, do you believe that Susan was bullied?

To answer this question, consider the following:

1. Question: Is this a repeated incident?
   Answer: No, as Susan has just returned from maternity leave.
2. Question: Was there a negative effect of the behaviour on Susan?
   Answer: Yes.
3. Question: Did Susan find it difficult to defend herself?
   Answer: Yes.
4. Question: Did the birthing unit coordinator intend to bully Susan?
   Answer: Unknown.

*Conclusion*: Bullying is not proven to have happened on this occasion. However, should another similar incident happen, bullying would be proven because it would be repeated and it would be likely there was intent.

**Box 2.5 Vignette: Disrespectful Behaviour in Front of a Woman and Birthing Person**

The following vignette is a true description of a newly qualified midwife, Hodan's (pseudonym) experience of caring for Amelia, who was in the second stage of labour, about to give birth to her second baby. Amelia's partner was supporting her and Hodan had developed a good relationship with both Amelia and her partner. Amelia was progressing well, there had been no complications, the vertex was visible and advancing slowly with each contraction. Hodan started to prepare for the birth when suddenly the door was flung open with no warning and the birthing unit coordinator marched into the room saying in a very load voice, 'This woman needs an episiotomy, have you got the local anaesthetic ready? Why haven't you done one already?' Hodan's legs turned to jelly, her heart rate increased and she became unable to say anything; *this coordinator had been present at her last two births and had criticised her in front of the woman and birthing person on both occasions.* The coordinator started to inform Amelia that Hodan was going to inject her with local anaesthetic and was going to perform an episiotomy. Amelia gave consent for this, but Hodan did not agree believing that there was no indication for an episiotomy, but did not want to argue in front of Amelia and her partner, so reluctantly performed the episiotomy after which Amelia gave birth to a baby girl. After the placenta had been born and the coordinator had left the room, Amelia turned to Hodan and said, 'thank goodness that midwife came into the room, she knew what she was doing'. Hodan's confidence was shattered, and she started to look at the off duty to see when she was working with the coordinator so that she could try and change her shifts.

> **Box 2.6 Exercise 2: Defining Bullying Behaviour**
> After reading the above vignette and by applying the defining attributes described above, do you believe that Hodan was bullied?
> To answer this question, consider the following:
>
> 1. Question: Is this a repeated incident?
>    Answer: Yes, this is the third time it has happened.
> 2. Question: Was there a negative effect of the behaviour on Hodan?
>    Answer: Yes.
> 3. Question: Did Hodan find it difficult to defend herself?
>    Answer: Yes.
> 4. Question: Did the birthing unit coordinator intend to bully Hodan?
>    Answer: Yes, probably.
>
> *Conclusion*: Bullying is likely to have happened on this occasion.

These criteria can be applied by any person who believes they or someone they know is being bullied and by any manager who is investigating an allegation of bullying.

## 2.7.5   The Detrimental Effects of Bullying Behaviour

The effects of being subjected to bullying behaviour can be devastating with lasting physiological, psychological and behavioural harm (Burleigh et al. 2023; Capper 2021; Oates et al. 2020; O'Brien 2018b; Gillen et al. 2008, 2009; RCM 1996, 2016). A member of staff who is being targeted will first become reluctant to work with the person who is targeting them. As a result, they will seek to change their shifts when they are rostered together. Then, they often go 'off sick' to avoid the person and may eventually go on long-term sick leave or leave the profession altogether (Burleigh et al. 2023; Ball et al. 2002; RCM 1996, 2016). As an RCM regional officer representing midwives who had been bullied, the most concerning effect (other than the devastating suicidal ideology) was the obsessive dwelling on the bully and seeking justice or revenge. One midwife said to me that *'I wake up thinking about her, I go to sleep thinking about her, she is under my skin'*.

**Psychological Effects**
1. Anxiety
2. Panic attacks, often on the way to work
3. Inability to go to work
4. Depression
5. Feeling of dread
6. Tearfulness
7. Suicidal ideology

**Physiological Effects**
1.  Headaches/migraine
2.  Sweating/shaking
3.  Feeling/being sick
4.  Irritable bowel
5.  Raised blood pressure and respiratory rate
6.  Inability to sleep
7.  Burnout
8.  Exhaustion


**Behavioural Effects**
1.  Becoming irritable
2.  Becoming withdrawn
3.  Becoming aggressive
4.  Absenteeism
5.  Increased consumption of tobacco/alcohol
6.  Obsessive dwelling on the bully and seeking justice or revenge


## 2.7.6   Definition of Discrimination and Harassment

Discrimination Law (Equality Act 2010) protects people against discrimination at work (Advisory, Arbitration and Conciliatory Service [ACAS] 2025). Discrimination means treating someone 'less favourably' than someone else, because of their 'protected characteristics', which are as follows:

- Age
- Disability
- Gender reassignment
- Marriage and civil partnership
- Pregnancy and maternity
- Race
- Religion or belief
- Sex
- Sexual orientation

Less favourable treatment can be anything that puts someone with a protected characteristic at a disadvantage, compared to someone who does not have that characteristic. There is no legal definition of 'putting someone at a disadvantage'. But it might include the following:

- Excluding someone from opportunities or benefits
- Making it harder for someone to do their job

- Causing someone emotional distress
- Causing someone financial loss

It can still be discrimination even if the less favourable treatment was not intended. For pregnancy and maternity, discrimination means treating someone 'unfavourably' because there is no need to compare with how someone else is treated (ACAS 2025).

Discrimination means treating a person with certain protected characteristics *less favourably*, whilst harassment is *unwanted behaviour* towards a person with the same protected characteristics as discrimination apart from pregnancy and maternity and marriage and civil partnership.

Harassment and bullying are often confused (ACAS 2025); bullying behaviour can be harassment if the perpetrator targets someone who has protected characteristics. Managers of employees who fail to take steps to prevent harassment or investigate complaints may be held liable for their unlawful actions and could be required to pay compensation to the victim, as could the individual who has committed the act of harassment. Awards for injury to feelings go up to £30,000 and, in exceptional cases, may exceed this. The award to compensate an individual for loss of employment because of harassment is uncapped. Harassment on any grounds may also be a criminal offence, which means that in some cases, harassment could become a police matter. The Equality Act (2010) also poses an additional duty on public sector bodies to ensure that they are taking steps to create an inclusive environment, and tackle inequality.

## 2.8    How Do You Know if You Are Working in a Compassionate Culture?

A sign you have a positive workplace culture is laughter. Just listen to how much laughter there is where you work. Laughter is a good sign of positivity. You can work hard and still enjoy your workday more. (Glenn 2019)

There are differing theories of compassion (see Sect. 4.3) (Strauss et al. 2016; Gu et al. 2017; West et al. 2017); in healthcare, the theory of compassion specifically has been developed principally by The Kings Fund (2025) led by Professor Michael West (West and Bailey 2022; West 2021; West et al. 2017; West and Chowla 2017). The theory of compassion identifies the four elements of compassion (West 2021, p. 3) as attending, understanding, empathising and helping.

1. *Attending*: Paying attention to the other, being present and noticing their suffering
2. *Understanding*: Understanding what is causing the other's distress, by making an appraisal of the cause, ideally through a listening dialogue with that person to achieve a shared understanding

3. *Empathising*: Having an empathetic response, mirroring the other's feelings, having a felt relation with the other's distress, without being overwhelmed by those feelings
4. *Helping*: Taking intelligent (thoughtful, wise and appropriate) action to help relieve the other's suffering

In compassionate cultures, most staff display these qualities; 'compassion binds us together, creates a sense of safety and interconnectedness and is a manifestation of love in an encompassing rather than exclusive sense' (West 2021, p. 1). Do you think you work in a compassionate workplace? If you can identify the following indicators, there is a strong possibility that you do (O'Brien 2018a, c).

*Inclusion of everyone, no matter who they are, matters* and are included in all social events, consultations, planning for change, meetings, etc.

*Physiological safety* where all staff feel safe to raise concerns; therefore, levels of safety and quality of care for staff and women and birthing people are higher with good clinical outcomes.

*Educated and skilled professional staff* are encouraged to undertake postgraduate training and there are regular clinical education days for all staff.

*Positive perceptions of midwifery and women and birthing people*: You will never hear staff criticising and talking judgementally about women and birthing people.

*Staff have few mental health and physical sickness days*: With low vacancy and turnover rates, with people wanting to work there, due to reputation, the lower vacancy rates mean less stress in clinical areas.

*Few complaints from women, birthing people and families*: When staff are valued and respected, this is usually reflected in the care that women and birthing people receive.

*Innovative and dynamic*: With changes to practice and policies as new evidence emerges, all staff are encouraged to be curious and implement evidence-based practice.

Theories of compassion are explored in depth later in the book (see Sects. 4.3 and 7.2) and the importance of compassion in healthcare is reflected in the vignette below from a user of the NHS.

**Box 2.7 Vignette: Experiencing What We Do 'From the Other Side': A Personal Reflection (Ellen Kitson-Reynolds)**

I unfortunately sustained an injury that required a trip to a minor injuries department between Christmas and New Year. Having been someone who prided themselves on not 'being a drain to health services', I found myself feeling vulnerable whilst in a state of significant pain, not being able to problem solve and not having access to the resources to self-manage. I do have a long-term condition that is managed through annual outpatient's appointments that I can control and I am in control within the appointment and the pre-preparation to attend in a meaningful way.

These appointments are in one large NHS Trust with multi-sites. I have experienced, and am used to, the culture at this Trust. I am treated in a professional manner, given an equal partnership in my treatment and care planning and know the routines and expectations. I feel safe and valued as a continued user of this service.

I accessed a minor injuries unit in a satellite hospital of a different large NHS Trust. During this appointment, I was treated with care and compassion, but was informed that I would need to attend a different site for surgical intervention due to the nature of the injury. My initial reaction was of dread because I thought I would have to attend one of the sites linked to this NHS Trust. This was alleviated by being immediately informed that it would be one of the other sites I would be attending. I had not experienced this other site before but felt reassured that I was not attending the other closer site. This was based upon my experiences of supporting a number of family members who had not been spoken to well, ignored and not been given support, information or attention that I would constitute as kind or compassionate care. This is not just my experience but that of the various family members also depending on the type of service accessed in that particular site. It is also based upon reputation and what is presented in the media. The media portrays a very negative view of the care and treatment provided by the NHS generally, and one would be forgiven, believing that the NHS is 'broken' when in reality there is so much greatness provided for all. The pubic expect the best and expect a duty of candour. We expect NHS Trusts to investigate, hold a mirror up to themselves and we expect aspects of care to be reviewed, changed and made better. However, when this happens, it appears that people are only interested in the negative and not the things that work well or are exceptional.

I attended my day-care surgical appointment and was introduced to a number of professionals from various professions. I was made to feel special and safe with every single person I came into contact with who was kind and compassionate. Each professional was wearing a theatre hat or name badge clearly visible with their name and profession. They all introduced themselves and spoke in professional and friendly ways, always smiling and appropriately happy. Although I felt I was a drain of the resources with the number of

(continued)

**Box 2.7**  (continued)

people, equipment and theatre space used for something of my own making [I was adding up the pound signs and thinking how much is this costing?], I was not in any way left feeling that this was an inconvenience or problem. I was aware that the current 'winter pressures' were at capacity in the region and that my attendance would be a compounding factor. This never was obvious in my care provision.

My experience has left me feeling proud of my fellow NHS colleagues and note what a fantastic role they play when they themselves may feel the pressures of the healthcare system. Personally, I am surprised at how emotional this experience left me. Vulnerability and pain are exhausting. The injuries or health issues people face can be significant, or not, in continuing with daily activities. Feeling out of control in an area that is unfamiliar to you can exacerbate these feelings. I am a healthcare professional and have insights into the NHS world. What must it be like for those who do not know how this all works. It is a very humbling reminder to experience what we do from the other side. It is good to remember these experiences so that others receive kind and compassionate best care when we are the care providers. It is also a reminder of how patient stories are shared within friendship and family groups and within the media. Perhaps I will no longer fear being a patient in the other NHS Trust site!

**Box 2.8 Exercise: What Is Your Response to a Distressed Midwife?**

Annie is a newly qualified midwife working on the birthing unit in a maternity unit in London. Whilst at work, she is called into the coordinators office and informed that the coordinator has been contacted by Annie's sister and informed that her father has been admitted to the intensive care unit in a hospital in Scotland. Figures 2.1 and 2.2 below give two possible immediate responses from the coordinator.

Please reflect on what your immediate response would be if you were the birthing unit coordinator?

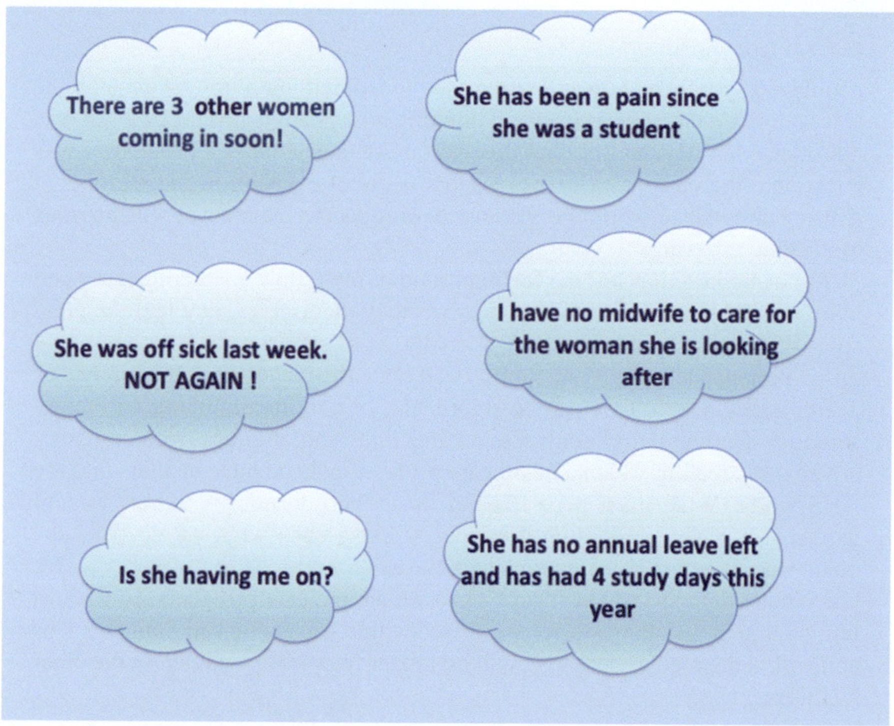


**Fig. 2.1** An example of a discompassionate culture

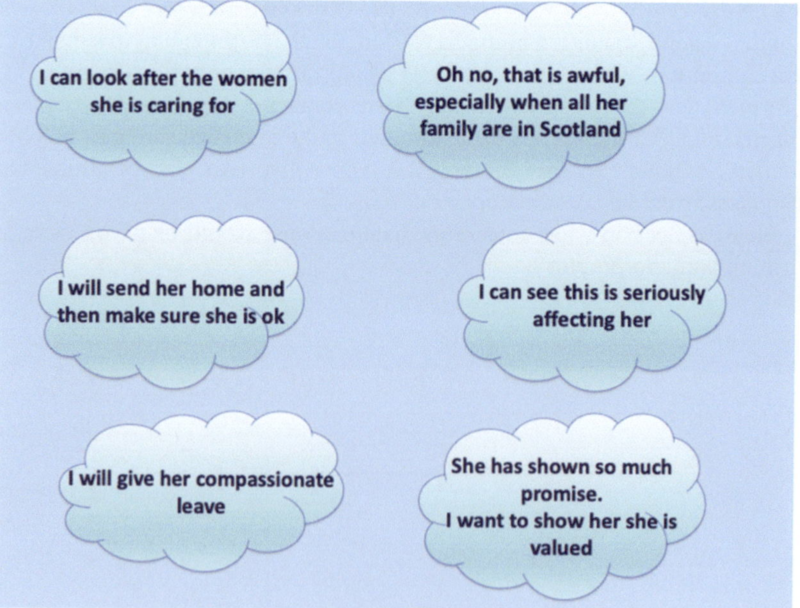


**Fig. 2.2** An example of a compassionate culture

## 2.9    Conclusion

This chapter has set the context and background for the remainder of the book by identifying 'where we are now' through examining research evidence and reports of maternity service reviews. It has looked at how cultures develop and flourish both positively and negatively, including effects of the 'tall poppy syndrome'. The differences between disrespectful and bullying behaviour are identified, with an exercise provided to test if you are able to identify the differences through the use of four defining attributes, determined through Gillen et al.'s (2004) concept analysis. The importance of achieving inclusion is demonstrated with kindness and compassion explored through the lens of women and birthing people. This chapter ends by explaining what a compassionate workplace looks like, asking if you believe you are currently working in one. Chapter 3 will go on to examine the stresses of the current workplace for maternity and neonatal staff, with remaining chapters drawing together the 'golden threads of change' (OED 2025) to look at different ways of resolution.

## References


Advisory, Arbitration and Conciliatory Service ACAS (2025) Discrimination and the Equality Act 2010. Available: https://www.acas.org.uk/discrimination-and-the-law (accessed 18 Feb 2025)

Ball L. Curtis P, Kirkham M (2002) Why do midwives leave? Royal College of Midwives: England

Begley C M (1999a) A study of student midwives' experiences during their two year education programme Midwifery (15);194–202

Begley C M (1999b) Student midwives' views of 'learning to be a midwife' in Ireland Midwifery (15); 264–273

Begley C M (2002) 'Great fleas have little fleas': Irish student midwives' views of the hierarchy in midwifery Journal of Advanced Nursing 38 (3):310–317

Burleigh A, Wylam J, Millar B, Gillen P, Webster J, McEwen K, Gayle E, Hughes D, Lawrie A (2023) #Saynotobullyinginmidwifery. Available: www.midwifery.org.uk/news/support/saynotobullyinginmidwifery-report/ (accessed 26 Jan 2025)

Byrom S, Downe S (2015) The roar behind the silence. Why kindness, compassion and respect matter in maternity care. Pinter & Martin Ltd., London, England

Capper T S, Thorn M, Muurlink O T (2022). Workplace violence in the Australian and New Zealand midwifery workforce: A scoping review. Journal of Nursing Management, 30(6): 1831–1842. Available: https://doi.org/10.1111/jonm.13766 (Accessed 26 Feb 2025)

Capper T 2021 Workplace bullying: The midwifery student experience [Online]. CQ University Australia. Available: https://acquire.cqu.edu.au/articles/thesis/Workplace_bullying_The_midwifery_student_experience/14776482/1/files/28395063.pdf (accessed 26 Jan 2025)

Care Quality Commission (2024) National Review of Maternity Services 2022 – 2024. Available: https://www.cqc.org.uk/publications/maternity-services-2022-2024 (accessed 5 Feb 2025)

Catling C, Reid F, Hunter B (2017) Australian midwives' experiences of their workplace culture. Women and Birth. 30(2):137–145 Available: https://doi.org/10.1016/j.wombi.2016.10.001 (Accessed 25 Feb 2025)

Catling C, Rossiter C (2020) Midwifery workplace culture in Australia: A national survey of midwives. Women and Birth 33: 464–472. Available: https://pubmed.ncbi.nlm.nih.gov/31676324/ (accessed 27 Jan 2025)

Commission for Healthcare Audit and Inspection (2006) Investigation into 10 Maternal Deaths, or Following Delivery at, North West London Hospitals NHS Trust between April 2002 and April

2005. London: England. Available: https://minhalexander.com/wp-content/uploads/2016/09/hcc-northwick-park-_tagged.pdf (accessed 26 Jan 2025)

Crowther C. (2020) Joy at Birth an Interpretive Hermeneutic, Phenomenological Inquiry. Routledge, UK

Curtis P, Ball L, Kirkham M (2003) Why do midwives leave? Talking to managers. London, England: Royal College of Midwives

Curtis P, Ball, L, Kirkham M (2006a). 'Bullying and horizontal violence: cultural or individual phenomena?' British Journal of Midwifery. 14(4A): 218–221 Available: https://shura.shu.ac.uk/252/ (accessed 28 Jan 2025)

Curtis P, Ball L, Kirkham M (2006b). 'Ceasing to practise midwifery: working life and employment choices'. British Journal of Midwifery. 14(6June): 336–338 Available: https://shura.shu.ac.uk/282/ (accessed 28 Jan 2025)

Curtis P, Ball L, Kirkham M (2006c) 'Flexible working patterns: balancing service needs or fuelling discontent?' British Journal of Midwifery. 14(5May): 260–262–264 Available: https://shura.shu.ac.uk/294/ (accessed 28 Jan 2025)

Curtis P, Ball L, Kirkham M (2006d) 'Working together? Indices of division within the midwifery workforce'. British Journal of Midwifery. 14(3March): 138–141 Available: https://shura.shu.ac.uk/335/ (accessed 28 Jan 2025)

Curtis P, Ball L, Kirkham M (2006e) 'Management and morale: challenges in contemporary maternity care'. British Journal of Midwifery. 14(2February): 100–103 Available: https://www.researchgate.net/publication/272544011_Management_and_morale_Challenges_in_contemporary_maternity_care (accessed 28 Jan 2025)

Curtis P, Ball L, Kirkham M (2006f). 'Why do midwives leave? (Not) being the kind of midwife you want to be'. British Journal of Midwifery, 14 (1 January): 27–29–31 Available https://shura.shu.ac.uk/323/ (accessed 28 Jan 2025)

Darzi, A. (2024) Independent Investigation of the National Health Service in England. Crown Copyright. Available: https://www.gov.uk/government/publications/independent-investigation-of-the-nhs-in-england (accessed 4 Feb 2025)

Department of Health (1993). Changing Childbirth: Report of the Expert Maternity Group Pt.1. London: HMSO

Donnison, J. (1988) Midwives and Medical Men. A history of the struggle for the Control of Childbirth 2nd edition, London: Historical Publications

Elliott M (2004) The RCM's New President Speaks Out. RCM Midwives Journal 7(6), p.232

Equality Act (2010) Legislation.govt.uk. Available at: https://www.legislation.gov.uk/ukpga/2010/15/contents (Accessed 20 Feb 2025)

Felker A, Patel R, Kotnis R, Kenyon S, Knight M (Eds.) on behalf of MBRRACE-UK. Saving Lives, Improving Mothers' Care Compiled Report – Lessons learned to inform maternity care from the UK and Ireland Confidential Enquiries into Maternal Deaths and Morbidity 2020-22. Oxford: National Perinatal Epidemiology Unit, University of Oxford 2024

Feeley C, Stacey T (2024) Novel solutions to the midwifery retention crisis in England: an organisational case study of midwives' intentions to leave the profession and the role of retention midwives. Midwifery. Available: https://doi.org/10.1016/j.midw.2024.104152 (accessed 28 Jan 2025)

Feeley C (2023) Skilled Heartfelt Midwifery Practice. Safe, Relational Care for Alternative Physiological Births. Springer, Switzerland Available https://doi.org/10.1007/978-3-031-43643-7 (accessed 7 Feb 2025)

Francis R (2013) Report of the Mid Staffordshire NHS Foundation Trust public inquiry: executive summary [online] The Stationary Office. Available: https://assets.publishing.service.gov.uk/government/uploads/system/uploads/attachment_data/file/279124/0947.pdf (accessed 26 Jan 2025)

Glenn S (2019) Does Laughter Belong in the Workplace? Available: https://www.samglenn.com/article/does-laughter-belong-workplace (Accessed 20 Feb 2025)

Gillen P, Sinclair M, Kernohan WG (2004) 'A concept analysis of bullying in midwifery'. Evidence Based Midwifery. 2(2):46–51. Available: https://pure.ulster.ac.uk/ws/portalfiles/portal/92266800/scan_e10047419_2021_09_16_15_58_48.pdf (accessed 28 Jan 2025)

Gillen P Sinclair M, Kernohan WG (2008) The nature and manifestations of bullying in midwifery. Belfast: Ulster University. Available: https://pure.ulster.ac.uk/ws/portalfiles/portal/101327391/Gillen_2008_bullying.pdf (accessed 26 Jan 2025)

Gillen P, Sinclair M, Kernohan GW, Begley C (2009) 'Student midwives' experience of bullying'. Evidence-Based Midwifery, 7(2):46+. Available: https://link.gale.com/apps/doc/A204894578/HRCA?u=anon~4ec74bf6&sid=googleScholar&xid=08e2bf29 (accessed 27 Jan 2025)

Gu J, Cavanagh K, Baer R, Strauss C. An empirical examination of the factor structure of compassion. PLoS One. 2017 Feb 17;12(2): e0172471. https://doi.org/10.1371/journal.pone.0172471. PMID: 28212391; PMCID: PMC5315311

Hadikin R, and O'Driscoll M (2000). The bullying culture: cause, effect, harm reduction. Books for Midwives Press, Oxford, England

Hunter B (2004) Conflicting ideologies as a source of emotion work in midwifery. Midwifery 20(3):261–271

Hunter, B. (2005) 'Emotion work and boundary maintenance in hospital-based midwifery', Midwifery Vol.21, pp.253–266

Hunter, B. (2010) 'Mapping the emotional terrain of midwifery: What can we see and what lies ahead?', Int. J. Work Organisation and Emotion, Vol. 3, No. 3, pp.253–269

Hunter B, Fenwick J, Sidebotham M, Henley J (2019). Midwives in the United Kingdom: Levels of burnout, depression, anxiety, and stress and associated predictors. Midwifery 79

Independent Maternity Review (2022) Ockenden report – Final: Findings, conclusions, and essential actions from the independent review of maternity services at the Shrewsbury and Telford Hospital NHS Trust (HC 1219) Crown. Available at https://assets.publishing.service.gov.uk/government/uploads/system/uploads/attachment_data/file/1064302/Final-Ockenden-Report-web-accessible.pdf (Accessed 9th Sept 2024)

Johnson J (2016) The lived experiences of student midwives subjected to inappropriate behaviour [Online]. University of Southampton. Available: https://eprints.soton.ac.uk/411282/1/Jane_Johnston_Thesis.pdf (accessed 28 Jan 2025)

Kirkham, M. (1999) 'The culture of midwifery in the National Health Service in England', Journal of Advanced Nursing Vol. 30, pp.732–739. Available: https://onlinelibrary.wiley.com/doi/10.1046/j.1365-2648.1999.01139 (accessed 1 Feb 2025)

Kirkup B (2022) Reading the signals, Maternity and Neonatal Services East Kent – the report of the independent investigation. London: His Majesty's Stationary Office. Available: https://assets.publishing.service.gov.uk/media/634fb083e90e0731a5423408/reading-the-signals-maternity-and-neonatal-services-in-east-kent_the-report-of-the-independent-investigation_print-ready.pdf (accessed 28 Jan 2025)

Kirkup B (2015) The Report of the Morecambe Bay Investigation. Available: http://data.parliament.uk/DepositedPapers/Files/DEP2015-0267/The_Report_of_the_Morecambe_Bay.pdf (Accessed 27 January 2025)

Kitson-Reynolds E (2010) The Lived Experience of Newly Qualified Midwives. Thesis, University of Southampton

Kitson-Reynolds E, Cluett E, Le-May A (2014) Fairy tale midwifery—fact or fiction: The lived experiences of newly qualified midwives. British Journal of Midwifery 22(9):660–668

Leap N (1997) 'Making sense of 'horizontal violence' in midwifery', British Journal of Midwifery. Vol. 5(11): 689

Maben J, Taylor C, Jagosh J, Carrieri D, Briscoe S, Klepacz N, Mattick K (2023) Delivering healthcare: a complex balancing act: A guide to understanding and tackling psychological ill-health in nurses, midwives and paramedics. University of Surrey, Guildford. www.workforceresearchsurrey.health

Mayra K, Catling C, Musa H, Hunter B, Baird K (2023) Compassion for midwives: The missing element in workplace culture for midwives globally. PLOS Glob Public Health 3(7): e0002034. https://doi.org/10.1371/journal.pgph.0002034

McAra-Couper J, Gilkison A, Crowther S, Hunter M, Hotchin C, Gunn J (2014). Partnership and reciprocity with women sustain Lead Maternity Carer midwives in practice. NZCOM Journal 49, 23–33. Available: https://doi.org/10.12784/nzcomjnl49.2014.5.29-33 (accessed 24 Feb 2025)

McNeil M, Kitson-Reynolds E (2024). Student midwives' experiences of clinical placement and the decision to enter the professional register. British Journal of Midwifery 32:14–20. Available: https://www.britishjournalofmidwifery.com/content/research/student-midwives-experiences-of-clinical-placement-and-the-decision-to-enter-the-professional-register/ (accessed 26 Jan 2025)

MSF Trade Union (1995) Bullying at work: how to tackle it. A Guide for MSF representatives and members. College Hill Press: London

NHS England (2016) Better Births: Improving Outcomes of maternity services in England. National Maternity Review. Available at https://www.england.nhs.uk/publication/better-births-improving-outcomes-of-maternity-services-in-england-a-five-year-forward-view-for-maternity-care/ (Accessed 9 Sept 2024)

NHS England (2022) Workforce, Training and Education. Available: https://www.hee.nhs.uk/our-work/quality/national-education-training-survey-nets/you-said-we-listened/583-student-midwives-considered-leaving-their-course-2022. Accessed 18 Feb 2025

NHS (2019). NHS Long Term Plan » Online version of the NHS Long Term Plan. [online] Longtermplan.nhs.uk. Available at: https://www.longtermplan.nhs.uk/online-version/. (Accessed: 29 November 2024)

Nursing and Midwifery Council (2019) Standards of Proficiency for Midwives. NMC, London Available: https://www.nmc.org.uk/globalassets/sitedocuments/standards/2024/standards-of-proficiency-for-midwives.pdf (Accessed 24 Feb 2025)

Oates J, Topping A, Watts K, Charles P, Hunter C, Arias T (2020) 'The rollercoaster': A qualitative study of midwifery students' experiences affecting their mental wellbeing. Midwifery 88. Available: https://doi.org/10.1016/j.midw.2020.102735 (accessed 5 Feb 2025)

Oxford English Dictionary (2025) Oxford University Press. Oxford Available at: https://www.oxfordlearnersdictionaries.com/definition/english/golden-thread?q=golden+thread (Accessed 28 Feb 2025)

O'Brien M (2018a) Developing a Compassionate Workplace. Presentation presented at the Northern Maternity and Midwifery Festival, Manchester. 26 June 2018

O'Brien M (2018b) Respectful Relationships in Maternity Services. Presentation presented at the Northern Maternity and Midwifery Festival. Manchester. 26 June 2018

O'Brien M (2018c) Practical Steps to Developing a Respectful and Caring Workplace: Challenging Bullying Behaviours. Presentation presented at Northern Maternity and Midwifery Festival. Cardiff. 20 Sept 2018

O'Brien M (2021) Case load practice and the national and international political/professional context. In E Kitson-Reynolds, and K Ashforth, (Eds) A Concise Guide to Continuity of Care in Midwifery (pp.18–33) London and New York: Routledge

Page L (2003) One-to-one Midwifery: Restoring the "With Woman" Relationship in Midwifery Journal of Midwifery & Women's Health 2003 Volume 48 (2):119–125

Royal College Midwives (1996) In place of fear: recognising and confronting the problem of bullying in midwifery RCM, London, England

Royal College Midwives (2016) Why midwives leave – revisited. RCM, London, England Available: https://cdn.ps.emap.com/wp-content/uploads/sites/3/2016/10/Why-Midwives-Leave (accessed 26 Jan 2025)

Royal College of Nursing (1996) Working Well: a call to employers. RCN: London

Sandall J (2017). The contribution of continuity of midwifery care to high quality maternity care, RCM

Sandall J, Charles P, Hunter C, Arias T (2016). "Midwife-led continuity models versus other models of care for childbearing women." Cochrane Database Syst Rev 4: CD004667

Sandall J (1997). Midwives' burnout and continuity of care. British Journal of Midwifery, 5(2), pp.106–111

Smith J (2021) Nurturing Maternity Staff. How to tackle trauma, stress and burnout to create a positive working culture in the NHS. Pinter and Martin, UK

Strauss C, Lever Taylor B, Gu J, Kuyken W, Baer R, Jones F, Cavanagh K. What is compassion and how can we measure it? A review of definitions and measures. Clin Psychol Rev. 2016 Jul;47:15–27. https://doi.org/10.1016/j.cpr.2016.05.004. Epub 2016 May 26. PMID: 27267346. Available: https://pubmed.ncbi.nlm.nih.gov/27267346/ (accessed 24 Feb 2025)

Tew, M. (1989). Safer Childbirth? A critical history of maternity care. London, Springer

The Kings Fund (2025) Available at https://www.kingsfund.org.uk/ (Accessed 20 Mar 2025)

Turner L (2021) Evidence base on case load held practice and outcomes. In E Kitson-Reynolds and K Ashforth (Eds) A Concise Guide to Continuity of Care in Midwifery. (pp 34–52) Routledge: 34–52

Verluysen M (1980) 'Old Wives Tales? Women Healers in English History' in C. Davies (ed.) Rewriting Nursing History. London, CroomHelm

West MA, Bailey S (2022) What is Compassionate Leadership. The Kings Fund https://www.kingsfund.org.uk/insight-and-analysis/long-reads/what-is-compassionateleadership (Accessed 25 Feb 2025)

West MA (2021) Compassionate Leadership: Sustaining Wisdom, Humanity and Presence Health and Social Care. London: Swirling Leaf Press

West M, Eckert R, Collins B, Chowla R, (2017) Caring to change: how compassionate leadership can stimulate innovation in health care 2017. The Kings Fund Available: https://assets.kingsfund.org.uk/f/256914/x/0b76247d02/caring_to_change_2017.pdf. (Accessed 24 Feb 2025)

West MA and Chowla R (2017) Compassionate leadership for compassionate health care. In P Gilbert (ed.), Compassion: Concepts, Research and Applications. Routledge, London, pp. 237–257. Available: https://doi.org/10.4324/9781315564296 Accessed 26 Feb 2022

Wylam (2023) Why do Newly Qualified and Student Midwives Leave. In A Barrett, A Burleigh, P Gillen, D Hughes (Eds.) #saynotobullyinginmidwifery (pp. 116–199). Available: www.midwifery.org.uk/news/support/saynotobullyinginmidwifery-report/ (accessed 26 Jan 2025)

# The Impact of Staffing Levels, Psychological Safety and Maternity Culture on Staff Behaviour

**3**

Lesley Turner and Jennifer Lancaster

## 3.1 Introduction

Inadequate staffing levels are very often given as the reason for disrespectful behaviour; through exploring evidence from both a national and international perspective, this chapter explores the impact of staffing levels, psychological safety and disrespectful cultures on staff behaviour. It is important to consider the context and contribution of work pressure. Behaviours should not be seen in isolation, but as part of the workplace culture, where each incident is different, and external factors may play a part in their origins. The pressure and environment may mean that small changes in behaviour evolve over time, without individuals necessarily being aware of this. Although inadequate staffing should not be seen as an excuse, it could contribute to coping behaviour, which is unprofessional and not aligned to team cohesion or growth. Furthermore, low staffing can also mean that leaders are *firefighting* rather than challenging disrespectful behaviour. To challenge behaviour would risk further conflict at a time when every staff member counts and is needed to run a service. The aspiration of having staffing levels, across all maternity services, is essential to providing psychological safety that enables maternity staff to provide high-quality care to women and neonates.

Although we see respectful, professional behaviour as essential, it is useful to explore the priorities in which care is delivered. When time is short, and demands are high, other areas such as safety should be considered first; however, problems arise when polite, constructive and inclusive communication does not occur. Additionally, in these circumstances, staff may lose sight of teamwork, interprofessional collaboration and kindness. It has been considered that compassion should be an 'always event' in maternity care, and that barriers to compassionate and

L. Turner · J. Lancaster (✉)
University of Southampton, Southampton, United Kingdom
e-mail: L.Y.Turner@soton.ac.uk; J.L.E.Lancaster@soton.ac.uk



M. O'Brien, E. Kitson-Reynolds (eds.), *Respectful Relationships in the Maternity Service*, https://doi.org/10.1007/978-3-032-04281-1_3

respectful behaviour need attention for the sake of families and maternity care staff (Coxon et al. 2024).

This chapter outlines the current staffing challenges, changes in workforce and models of midwifery care, working conditions and available evidence that maternity staff behaviour could be the result of one or more of these factors. It will explore the nature of midwives' work and particular stressors within it, coping cultures, blame, psychological safety and the impact on performance. Whilst the staffing crisis in midwifery is not new, the concerns over safety, and links between staffing shortages and adverse outcomes means it is now more important than ever to understand the extent of these impacts. Exposure to disrespectful behaviour has been linked with safety critical outcomes for service users (Civility Saves Lives 2024). Understaffing may be fuelling poor behaviour in maternity settings, which can lead to poor outcomes for the workforce itself, and an untold impact on midwifery attrition and mental health. The impact on students and newly qualified midwives will also be explored, as they are the key to making a long-lasting change in disrespectful organisational culture and associated staff behaviour.

## 3.2    The Nature of the Job

Midwifery is a physically and emotionally demanding occupation. It is a vocation that attracts personalities that are empathetic in nature, with a caring disposition and desire to be physically and emotionally present with women and pregnant people (Greenstock 2023). Whilst this makes midwives ideal candidates as autonomous practitioners for the life-changing nature of the perinatal period, it also makes them vulnerable to the multiple workplace complexities of the maternity services. Midwives want to be able to provide quality care that is woman-centred, and where organisational barriers to effective care are not part of every day. Childbirth has become progressively medicalised, with women and pregnant people requiring midwifery care that is more complex (Healy et al. 2016). This comes at a time when austerity has been imposed on public services over the previous 10 years (Darzi 2024) and reductions in staffing have been insisted upon as part of senior managers' targets. Not only does medicalisation often result in the provision of high-risk intrapartum and postnatal care, require additional decision making and emergency management, but it has also resulted in an increase in critical incidents (Adriaenssens et al. 2015). Where adverse events result in an investigation, midwives have reported feelings of perceived low self-efficacy, as though they are professionally damaged, particularly if continuing to work clinically where the incident took place. At this time, they require confidential support from organisational cultures that prioritise the well-being of its staff (Robertson and Thomson 2016). When these needs are not prioritised through the behaviour and actions of management and support networks, as is often the case (Alexander et al. 2021; Peyman et al. 2017; Sheen et al. 2016), this can increase the vulnerability to midwives' physical and psychological health. Furthermore, when midwives are encouraged to accomplish their increased workloads through effective task and time management, it can often lead to the need for perfectionism in their approach (Carvajal et al. 2024), which is intensified when an incident has occurred (Sheen et al. 2016; Bogren et al. 2020). Work-related stress, burnout and psychological ill-health are being increasingly associated with the nature of midwifery work, with the organised structure of midwifery care exacerbating the personal risk (Maben et al. 2023).

With the shift in the medical needs of the pregnant person, and the recent reports and investigations into maternity services in the United Kingdom (UK), attention is on safety and the need for a more effective healthcare system for the perinatal population and the staff it represents. Amid a staffing crisis, National Health Service (NHS) organisations must be seen to be addressing these very real concerns if maternity care is to change for the better. Improvements need to be seen at all levels, from the government's response to the independent report into the health service (Darzi 2024) and subsequent launch of the national conversation towards reform (Department of Health and Social Care [DHSC] 2024), to the structured well-being support that is offered to maternity staff. Understanding and acknowledging the extent of the challenges are the start of being able to implement effective solutions.

## 3.3    Staffing Challenges

The value of midwifery has been noted globally, and the presence of midwives is claimed to contribute to over 56 health and well-being measures for mothers and babies (Renfrew et al. 2014). There is an international shortage of approximately 900,000 midwives and this is linked to extreme consequences in low- to middle-income countries. Midwives have a key role in preventing and reducing neonatal and maternal mortality, and it is projected that 2.2 million deaths could be averted by 2035 if midwifery provision was scaled up in the 88 most affected countries (Nove et al. 2021). It is estimated that the UK alone is short of 2500 midwives (Bonar 2019). An unsurprising impact of this is an increased workload for midwives, with recent estimates totalling 100,000 unpaid hours worked each week (Royal College of Midwives [RCM] 2022a). The Royal College of Nursing (RCN) undertook an NHS Staff Survey, demonstrating that only 29% of nurses and midwives said there was enough staff to do their job properly and 46% had felt unwell due to work-related stress (RCN 2024).

The staffing challenges relate not only to the number of midwives in the population (midwifery density) but also the increasing complexity of care required by ante-natal, intra-partum and postnatal women and neonates. The most recent figures in England show that the caesarean section rate is now 38% and the instrumental birth rate is 11% (NHS Digital 2023). The rate of induction of labour has risen following recommendations to induce women with post-dates pregnancies at the earlier gestation of 39 weeks. In a cross-sectional survey of 71 maternity units in England, the average induction rate was 36% of women, ranging from 19% to 52% (Taylor et al. 2024). The fast pace of admissions and discharges to maternity units is associated with increased rates of harmful incidents, errors and delays (Turner et al. 2024) and this element of workload has not been addressed to date. When wards are understaffed in the preceding week, this is associated with increased sickness absence in nurses, showing that adverse working conditions have consequences for staff as well as service users (Dall'Ora et al. 2024).

### 3.3.1  Staff Retention and Vacancies

Retaining staff is less costly and a faster way of maintaining the workforce than waiting for new recruits to qualify (Moncrieff et al. 2023). Retention also contributes to long-term stability rather than having a 'revolving door' workforce, which is constantly in a state of flux. The Reducing Pre-registration Attrition and Improving Retention project (Health Education England 2018) has scrutinised factors causing attrition of staff, throughout the student journey and during the first 2 years after registration. Predominant factors include financial strain and lack of placement support for students, and difficult transition to qualified roles for new registrants. This is important to tackle as students and early-career staff are at particular risk of leaving (Kinman et al. 2020).

Best practice for optimising retention has been shared, and some organisations have now employed 'retention midwives' with the aim of supporting early-career staff (Feeley and Stacey 2024). One model involves late-career staff remaining in the service as a *legacy mentor* (NHS England 2024a). It is important that older midwives are not lost from the workforce, due to not only their numbers but also the experience and wisdom that they bring. The average retirement age for midwives is 58.1 years, and currently, 41% of midwives are over 50 years (RCM 2022b; Taylor et al. 2022). Apart from retirement, the most common reasons for midwives leaving the profession are workload and staffing (44%) and disillusionment with the quality of care they can provide (27%) (Nursing and Midwifery Council [NMC] 2019).

Organisations are finding it hard to fill vacancies as 77% of Heads of Midwifery (HOMs) reported that recruiting experienced midwives was difficult or very difficult (RCM 2022b). Almost three quarters (72%) of HOMs are calling in bank or agency staff nearly every day as noted in the Manthorpe and Baginsky's (2023) review on midwives' morale, retention and recruitment. Recent moves to improve staffing have involved the recruitment of international educated midwives in the hope that they will be retained long term and progress in their careers (Manthorpe and Baginsky 2023).

Studies focussing on the positive aspects of retention are starting to be published, examining why midwives remain in their jobs despite the challenges (Bloxsome et al. 2019; Moncrieff et al. 2023). Valuing working relationships, building relationships with women and a passion for midwifery are some elements that midwives stayed in their roles for. Highlighting these positive aspects is particularly welcome after the COVID-19 pandemic and its impact on work patterns and well-being of staff (Stockdale 2023).

### 3.3.2  The Model of Midwifery Care and Organisation of Staff

The way midwives are organised, their level of autonomy and resources to do their job well also impact their well-being. Some amount of challenge is healthy, although the number of tasks and ever-increasing 'tick boxes' can mean that staff can feel overwhelmed in such a fast-paced environment. Continuity models of care may be protective against burnout, but in some cases, heavy workloads and the unpredictable nature of work can have a personal cost (Turner 2021). Relational models are thought to nurture compassion, as the women know the midwives caring for them and vice versa, facilitating mutual communication and trust (Mayra et al. 2023). Sufficient staffing levels are needed to implement continuity of career, and in some areas, shortages of staff have led to resentment between teams, which has been a barrier to implementation (McCourt et al. 2023) (see Sect. 2.5).

Shortages of staff mean that midwives are sometimes redeployed to cover other areas of the maternity service at short notice. This contributes to a state of unsteadiness which has been described as 'unexpected unmooring' and a sense of depersonalisation. This is described in the thesis by Spence (2023) entitled *I'm just a number, I'm not a person*. Anxiety is generated when the needs of the organisation and efficiency are prioritised. One participant said, *'You don't know where you're going to get pulled to, so you can't really sort of mentally prepare'* (Spence 2023, p. 173). Movement of staff can affect the cohesion of teams and the potential for mistrust and miscommunication in newly formed groups. Stable influencers in the workforce may no longer be present, which may lead to heightened tension and risks to psychological safety. A study by Hope et al. (2022) found that patients find it difficult to ask for help if the staff appear to be distracted or dismissive. A similar phenomenon may also be occurring for staff moving between areas at times of heightened activity, and group dynamics may be affected.

## 3.4  The Working Culture

Where the staffing constraints, operational environments and organisation of care delivery negatively impact working conditions and the perception of these challenges becoming normalised, the development of a coping culture evolves. A coping culture does not promote vulnerability or encourage team cohesion. It normalises vulnerable circumstances as acceptable:

> The culture in many maternity organisations normalizes secrecy, silences staff, and responds with judgement, usually in the form of 'that's just the way it is, and you just need to get on with it'. This culture is not conducive to optimizing staff mental wellbeing. (Smith 2021, p. 87)

The notion of a coping culture is further exacerbated by the responsibility of psychological well-being sitting with individual staff members, with emphasis on participating in mindfulness, prioritising patient outcome over experience, and where access to support services is only realistically achievable in the staff members' own time (Greenstock 2023). This personal responsibility for processing and adapting to the working environment is replicated within the concept of resilience (See Sect. 3.8) In discussion with Jan Smith (2021), Amity Reed, author of Overdue (Reed 2020), describes how the system is failing all of those involved in the experience of birth:

> Every time I saw our inhumane working conditions normalized… a small piece of my bright, beating heart was chipped away. Much of what I had learned at university and from my employer and union over the years about managing stress and trauma in midwifery was about building resilience and practicing self-care. Reminders to go for walks, talk to a friend or colleague, practice yoga or meditation and enjoy some downtime to decompress were all around me. I internalized these messages to the point where I felt responsible for my own ability to adapt to and accept the system I worked in. (Smith 2021, p. 65)

The lack of staffing and medical complexity of women is directly associated with increased time constraints on midwives. Time is a commodity that is prioritised for clinical tasks and documentation, with midwives reporting less availability to be 'with women' or to deliver the personalised quality aspect of care. With restricted time, teams are often not able to participate in activities that promote cohesion and productivity, such as introductions and familiarisation with fellow team members, huddles to discuss potential internal and external stressors and debriefing to process events that have the potential to be traumatic (Geraghty et al. 2019). In addition, time constraints and the working environment have a documented impact on an inability to meet the physiological needs of midwives. The basic physical needs of staff including breaks, food and hydration, and use of the toilet are often reported as lacking in much of the literature (Ford 2020).

Where the working culture and ability to practise being 'with woman' are at a discord, midwives are often left to internalise the impact. This can lead to moral injury, where the human connection is lost within our care (Newnham and Kirkham 2019). This is demonstrated through the work of Geraghty et al. (2019).

> Many participants cited specific incidents, including obstetric interventions … that involved over-seeing trauma occur to women during the childbirth process. (Geraghty et al. 2019, p. 302)

The psychological impact of moral injury includes feelings of guilt, shame and frustration. Subsequent behavioural impacts can vary, including social distancing, substance misuse and avoidance activities such as overworking (Greenstock 2023). Similarly, the stress that is often associated with poor working cultures and moral injury has also been linked to poor sleep or insomnia, harmful behaviours such as excessive eating and unexplained pain or painful symptoms, which are often the initial bodily response (Spencer 2015).

### 3.4.1  Do Staff Report Behavioural Incidents and Low Staffing Levels?

Staff are encouraged to report incidents of unprofessional behaviour that they either witness or experience themselves. There are certainly mechanisms to do this within organisations via incident report forms, senior leadership meetings, unions, student evaluations, listening events, civility champions and via Freedom to Speak Up Guardians. While under-reporting is likely, there has been a 28% increase in incidents notified to the Freedom to Speak Up Guardians in 2023–2024, compared to the previous year (National Guardian Office 2024). Inappropriate attitudes or behaviours were the most common themes, accounting for two in five reports (19.8%).

Some staff may be deterred from reporting incidents for fear that they may not be believed; they may feel shame or be afraid of potential repercussions (Hoel et al. 2007). Another aspect is whether the person is likely to feel heard or how confident they are that action will take place. This lack of accountability is described as 'organisational deafness' (Aunger et al. 2023). Creese et al. (2024) explore this further and note the disconnect and distance between clinicians and their managers. In this study, staff spoke about having concerns dismissed or denied, summed up in the title of their paper *They say they listen. But do they really listen?*

Low staffing levels should be reported as incidents, regardless of whether clinical harm has resulted from this. It is helpful to detail the care that was left undone or incomplete as a result, and not to accept that low staffing levels are a normal event and therefore unremarkable. Staffing data are presented at hospital board level in NHS Trusts and are also scrutinised during Care Quality Commission (CQC) inspections (CQC 2021). An example where a nurse campaigned tirelessly to expose understaffing, culture and quality issues is the example of Helene Donnelly who contributed to the Mid Staffordshire Public Inquiry (Crown Prosecution 2011). She completed over 50 incident reports and raised concerns verbally with managers, but felt her concerns were ignored. A climate of fear prevented other staff reporting the issues. Since this time, it is commonplace for whistleblowing policies to be shared with staff, with the expectation that they will speak up about anything that impacts patient care or their working lives. Under this arrangement, staff can disclose details without fear of detrimental treatment or reprisals. The Safe Learning Environment Charter helps students to understand positive expectations from the work environment and enables them to highlight areas where improvements are needed within a common framework (NHS England 2024b). Both staff and students should feel safe to raise concerns, for the sake of fellow colleagues and families in their care.

## 3.5    The Pressure Cooker: Does the Work Environment Contribute to Disrespectful Behaviour?

Repeated exposures to incidents can lead to compassion deficit in some midwives, where they become insensitive to the feelings of others (Spence 2023). Lack of compassion was noted in the report of the failings in the Mid Staffordshire Trust (Francis 2013), Morcambe Bay (Kirkup 2015) and Shewsbury and Telford (Ockenden 2022). It is argued by Spence (2023) that the workload pressure experienced by midwives perpetuates the *conveyor belt* pattern of work. Midwives are striving to give high-quality personalised care, and being unable to provide this level of care is counter to their inherent values. The COVID-19 pandemic magnified the staffing crisis, bringing it to the fore (Cordey et al. 2022). The early part of the pandemic was characterised by camaraderie and strong teamwork; however, this did not last as unmanageable workloads led to poor morale, compassion fatigue and moral distress. Strong working relationships are a protective factor against stress; however, negative working relationships add to the pressure (Cull et al. 2020). Burnout is multifactorial, but has been associated with high job demands, low control and low levels of support (Adriaenssens et al. 2015).

Aunger et al. (2023) found that key contributors to unprofessional behaviour included workplace frustration and disempowerment, cultures that tolerate unprofessional behaviour, poor social cohesion, inability to speak up and managers who appear unaware or unresponsive to these difficulties. Staff may engage in negative workplace behaviours to release feelings of frustration about negative job characteristics; shift patterns (12-h shifts) are associated with exhaustion, reduced coping and compromised emotional regulation. These factors could be linked to reduced compassion and self-protection behaviours (Rydon-Grange 2018). It is disappointing to see that less than one-third of midwives in an Australian study felt they worked in a positive culture (Catling and Rossiter 2020). Excessive workloads, time pressure and poor communication left midwives feeling despondent and disempowered. A study in Germany found that staff shortages hindered safe communication between maternity professionals (Schmiedhofer et al. 2021). Physical and emotional exhaustion can lead to symptoms of detachment. It is clear from UK and international literature that challenging work environments contribute to toxic cultures and incivility, and junior members of staff are most affected (Mayra et al. 2023).

## 3.6    The Importance of Psychological Safety, a 'Golden Thread of Change' (OED 2025)

The foundation of the NMC values originates from fair and kind behaviours, where relationships and best practice work together to promote excellence in nursing and midwifery (NMC 2020). Despite this, the recent Independent Culture Review of the Nursing and Midwifery Council Workplace (2024) outlined a history of concerns regarding the culture within the regulatory body itself. Fear of implications and a lack of confidence in organisational behaviour change prevented staff from speaking out (see Sect. 3.4.1). Furthermore, the report highlighted incidents of bullying and poor behaviours, failures in leadership and a *hostile and demoralising work environment* (NMC 2024, p. 86). This clear disregard for role-modelling professionalism is concerning; it is the role of the NMC to be seen to be demonstrating its own values, acting as a role model to the professionals it regulates. When the behaviour of leaders is contradictory to the values they represent, this questions accountability and damages trust (James-Edwards 2023). Nazir Afzal, the solicitor tasked with completing the review of the governing body for midwives, highlights the importance of workplace culture as a determinant of performance, outcomes, behaviour and professional development of staff within it. This review demonstrates the crucial nature of workplace culture on creating an environment of support and candour in safeguarding service users: *Toxic and unsafe environments create stress and fear for staff, which takes more energy and is depleting* (Smith 2021, p. 49). Another example of a loss of trust and respect due to lack of integrity amongst its leaders is Boris Johnson's repeated negligence of the COVID-19 regulations made by his own government, demonstrating a *failure of leadership* (Gray 2022). Both high-profile examples of poor leadership are examples of failure to create psychological safety within the NMC and the government with far-reaching consequences.

Fear negatively impacts learning and collaboration, essential components for maternity care that is increasingly multidisciplinary. This divergence was demonstrated within the Ockenden Report (2022), whereby a *them and us* culture between maternity disciplines was reported as damaging for psychological safety. Psychological safety supports individual risk-taking within a team, allowing staff members to vocalise thoughts, ideas and concerns without fear of retribution (Edmondson 2018). Feeling fearful impairs the working memory, analytical thinking and the ability to problem-solve. For NHS Trusts where hierarchy is evident, lower status is linked to stress and fearful behaviours. These behaviours have been linked to incivility, as stress can cause impatience and diminish communication. This directly impacts teamwork, the importance of which is described by Kivimaki et al. (2001) (cited in Smith 2021, p. 90): *Poor teamwork is the most significant contributor to absenteeism in medical staff.*

When evaluating working culture (see Sect. 3.6), it is important to consider the structure of teams in midwifery. Midwifery care within the UK is often delivered within a rostered system. A recent NHS Staff Survey (NHS England 2021) identified that over half of midwives' working patterns feature changeable pseudo teams, reflecting the 24/7 shiftwork aspect of the role. As humans, we have a need for relationships and to feel as though we belong (West 2012; Smith 2021). These needs are challenged when the nature of the job requires interdependent working as part of flexible teams, and commitment to a working schedule that is system focused. This has implications for psychological safety, with greater disconnect and a lack of trust and inclusion, fewer opportunities for feedback and encouragement and feelings of impersonal belonging can prevail (West 2021). This is further challenged by the often-adopted organisational approach of encompassing all staff as 'one team'. From a practical perspective, pseudo teams are associated with increased professional errors, fragmented care and staff absenteeism (West 2012). This high-lights the importance of professional relationships, as depersonalisation generates an absence of psychological safety (Greenstock 2023).

The working culture of an organisation impacts the likelihood of midwives asking for help. A culture that allows bullying to occur emphasises power and creates an environment where midwives are reluctant to reach out and ask questions or seek support due to fear of intimidation or humiliation (Cull et al. 2020). Conversely, a psychologically safe work environment supports those within it to share concerns, mistakes, and to ask questions:

> Psychological safety is essential for communicating, collaborating, experimenting, and ensuring the well-being of others in a wide variety of team and organisational settings. (Edmondson 2018, p. 28)

The consequences for speaking up and asking for help are positive, with no risk of humiliation, being ignored or apportion of blame. A mutual respect exists between colleagues, enabling effective collaboration across disciplines (Edmondson 2018). Harnessing and facilitating psychological safety within the changing context of the maternity environment promote the value of contribution from individual staff, the learning that can be gained from prompt reporting of adverse events (Frese and Keith 2015), and is essential for high performance in what leadership and organisational learning expert Amy Edmondson (2018, p. 26) terms as Volatile Uncertain Complex and Ambiguous (VUCA) conditions, such as healthcare.

Midwives are aware of the importance of learning from incidents when striving for better, safer maternity care, and value opportunities to do so (Carvajal et al. 2024). A culture that supports continual learning from events without judgement improves the quality of learning (Love et al. 2017). As Edmondson (2018) reports, when psychological safety exists, staff speak up and report errors, participating in learning behaviours. When leadership promotes candour and values the interdependent nature of the complex patient, teams are less likely to make errors but are also more inclined to report them. The evidence shows that understaffing is associated with increased adverse incident reporting (Turner et al. 2024). The handling of adverse events is linked to the level of psychological safety within an organisation (see Sect. 3.4.1). When staff are supported to uphold safety, when their views are actively listened to, when their hands are held during the management of an incident and the opportunity for learning is considerate of the feelings of those involved, the risk of staff trauma is reduced (Smith 2021). Considering the current understaffing climate, supporting a psychologically safe culture in maternity is crucial: 'candor, transparency and learning from error—a psychological safety triad' (Edmondson 2018, p. 111). As with learning from errors, when staff have the freedom to fail and are encouraged to accept failure as an integral part of learning and innovation, this is reflective of professional development and improvements to the quality of care. What is clear is that leadership that actively supports psychological safety is essential for failures to come to light (Edmondson 2018) and therefore be addressed, with the principal goal of achieving high-quality maternity services.

## 3.7 Leadership: Navigating the Challenges

Ineffective leadership has been repeatedly highlighted by the CQC recent Trust inspections as a significant contributor to the poor maternity working environment and subsequent staffing concerns (Wyeman 2024). The foundation of leadership is focused on coordinating the efforts of others to achieve as a collective what cannot be achieved as an individual (Edmondson 2018). It is the responsibility of the leader to appropriately assess the knowledge and skills of the individual members of the team when allocating task responsibility. Successful leaders demonstrate the ability to use emotional intelligence to support the psychological and physiological needs of the team members. Effective communication and linguistic skills support a leader to motivate and encourage team members, providing positive feedback and guidance on performance (Hearns 2022). Leadership within volatile uncertain complex and ambiguous (VUCA) conditions (Edmondson 2018) that is inclusive of the team's perspectives demonstrates flexibility, humility and vulnerability (Hearns 2022).

Creating a positive working culture begins with leaders, and, as Jan Smith describes in her work on *Nurturing Maternity Staff* (2021), this is the responsibility of everyone and can be demonstrated through all forms of interactions with colleagues. Quality leadership is also essential for maintaining a positive workplace culture (NMC 2024). Leaders at all levels within an organisation are responsible for creating and maintaining psychological safety, a dynamic and ongoing process that prioritises the importance of working culture (Edmondson 2018). Vulnerability as a leader is essential in a culture of psychological safety. Vulnerability itself is a courageous act of uncertainty and encourages the development of connections (Brown 2015), trust and authenticity (Hearns 2022). Demonstrating humility promotes team engagement in learning, discourages the perception of hierarchy and role-models professional performance behaviours. For example, when experiencing cognitive overload, leaders who reach out to the team for support in decision making and task completion are promoting team performance. Furthermore, this can result in cognitive reframing from the perspective of the leader, encouraging a team approach to address challenges whilst acknowledging individual input. When reflecting on adverse incidents, effective leaders engage in honest discussions and are emotionally expressive (Hearns 2022). Coyle (2018) describes how this form of role modelling can have beneficial effects on organisational culture. Through active vulnerability and humility, a leader can create a supportive culture of openness, enhancing the safety and well-being of staff and patients (see Boxes 3.1 and 3.2).

**Box 3.1 Vignette: Conflicting Priorities**
Madeline* (pseudonym) had been qualified as a midwife for 3 years. Having completed her training and preceptorship programme, Madeline took the decision to join one of the Trust's continuity of care midwifery teams. Whilst carrying a caseload within the continuity team, Madeline was also required to be a part of the Trust's contingency response, should the midwifery staffing not meet the needs of the maternity service users.

(continued)

**Box 3.1** (continued)

Following the COVID-19 pandemic, and during a period of increased sickness and absenteeism amongst the midwifery staff, the continuity team midwives were increasingly relied upon as contingency. As a result, Madeline was finding it difficult to balance the complex care needs of the women and pregnant people on her caseload with the increased hours spent staffing the unit, in addition to a balance with her personal life.

Fearing for the safety of the women on her caseload, who were already deemed vulnerable as part of the continuity care criteria, Madeline raised her concerns with senior staff members. Feeling as though her concerns were not heard, Madeline continued to feel as though the women in her care were being let down. The situation persisted until Madeline's feeling of despair turned into disconnect from the job. The challenges of battling safe staffing with a caseload, a lack of managerial support, with failed attempts at a work–life balance became too much, and Madeline decided to leave the profession, creating another vacancy within the workforce.

**Box 3.2 Vignette: The Impact on Midwives' Health and Well-Being of Providing Fragmented Care**

As part of her preceptorship, Michelle* (pseudonym) was required to rotate between the maternity wards within the Trust, completing the band five competencies and developing her confidence as an autonomous practitioner. With an increase in sickness and absenteeism in the midwifery workforce since the COVID-19 pandemic, Michelle's preceptorship was impacted by staffing shortages and redeployment.

With an increased requirement for midwives on the delivery suite, Michelle found that she spent the majority of her shifts as a newly qualified midwife providing 1:1 labour and birth care. Although this enabled her to develop her intrapartum skills and experience, Michelle found that it was increasingly challenging to complete her competencies as a band five midwife in this environment (for example, finding an available midwife to supervise suturing).

With staffing an ongoing issue, experienced midwives with better time and task management were allocated multiple women who were not long postnatal, with the labour care being assigned to those with less experience. With 1:1 care at a premium, once baby had been born, care of these women was often handed over, freeing up that midwife to provide labour care in another room.

Michelle was disappointed at the inability to continue to be 'with woman' once birth had occurred and was concerned about the impact this was having on the women in her care. Furthermore, with the increasing complexity of the women on delivery suite and the ongoing staffing shortages, Michelle was required to care for women with comorbidities that she had little experience of, exacerbating the feelings of inadequacy and anxieties around safety.

(continued)

**Box 3.2**  (continued)

After a period of time, Michelle started to experience symptoms of burnout, compassion fatigue and moral injury. Having voiced her feelings to members of the senior team, and subsequently taking a short period of leave, knowing the pressures that the service was under, Michelle was keen to return. Michelle was determined to provide 'good' care, rotating through the antenatal and postnatal wards, clinging to the 'good' shifts.

Despite her best efforts, and love for midwifery, Michelle continued to feel like being a midwife was less about being 'with woman,' as her training had taught her, and more about completing a series of 'tick box' actions. To continue to be a midwife would mean ignoring her own thoughts, feelings and values, which was having a negative impact on her physical and mental health. Michelle made the difficult decision to prioritise her own well-being and leave midwifery, although still experiences grief at the loss of being a midwife.

For a typical shift, the initial allocation of tasks or workload is a core responsibility of the leader or midwife in charge. Leaders have oversight of workload planning and task prioritisation, based on the duration, urgency and interdependent nature of the tasks. This needs to be effectively delegated to the staff available, or the team of that shift. Confounding factors to the success of this action include awareness of team member skill, capabilities and experience, the correlation of the skill mix of available staff and managing expectations of the team (Hearns 2022). This can be challenging when you consider the junior nature of the midwifery workforce (NMC 2023) and the reality of pseudo teamworking.

It is easy to see how under the pressurised working conditions leadership can become task-focused rather than person-centred, despite the detrimental consequences to the workforce. Cummings et al. (2018) carried out a systematic analysis of leadership style and subsequent outcomes within nursing. They concluded that leadership that is focused on workload and not the relationship with staff members negatively impacts job satisfaction, productivity and ultimately staff attrition. Furthermore, leadership that is proactive and compassionate is significant in making staff feel supported following adverse events, mitigating feelings of abandonment and promoting value (Christoffersen et al. 2020). Midwives enter the profession where the purpose of caring and being able to make a difference to the lives of the women, service users and families is the motivation. However, when this motivation and ability to meet their needs is tested through extrinsic pressures, it falls to the leaders to emphasise a sense of purpose when navigating the stressors. Irrespective of the situation or individual experience, reminding staff of the meaning behind their efforts and offering praise reinforce their value (Bimpong et al. 2019; Hearns 2022; NHS England 2023b).

## 3.8    Performance when Under Pressure

The documented pressures that impact midwives' performance can be classified as intrinsic and extrinsic. Intrinsic pressures are task-related, whereas extrinsic pressures are the conditions in which the task is performed. Therefore, performance is both individual and a consequence of the environment (Hearns 2022). These elements can work together to modify our perception of pressure. Psychologists have identified four states of performance: disengagement, flow, frazzle and freeze or choking (Csikszentmihalyi 1990; Goleman 2011). Flow is the ultimate state of performance, where pressure and capability are equal; the situation is challenging, but can be successfully addressed with the *'knowledge, skills and resources to achieve a safe and favourable outcome'* (Hearns 2022, p. 2).

Staff engagement is significant in healthcare, with disengagement leading to safety concerns and staff turnover (Edmondson 2018). Recent studies have explored the relationship between psychological safety and engagement, with healthcare staff reporting having trust in management (Chughtai and Buckley 2013), supportive relationships with colleagues (May et al. 2004) and commitment to the organisation as enhancing engagement. In addition to this, an increase in stressors and decrease in the ability to be 'with woman' negatively impact staff commitment and engagement (Geraghty et al. 2019). Feeling able to provide safe care has also been linked to engagement (Rathert et al. 2009). This raises further concerns considering the connection between midwives participating in what they believe to be poor care and the associated feelings of trauma (Smith 2021; Greenstock 2023), and the increase in moral injury as a result of midwives' external constraints being prioritised over the founding midwifery principle of being 'with woman' (Greenstock 2023, p. 40). It is important to consider the cognitive and behavioural impact of the pressures at play in the maternity environment to gain an understanding of the physical and psychological consequences midwives experience. Midwives perceive pressure by evaluating risk and the ability to address the situation. Whilst this cognitive appraisal takes time, an emotional assessment occurs much faster, providing an emotional response. If the brain recognises the pressure as one previously experienced, the physiological and psychological response is likely to result in a flow performance state. However, if the appraisal is of threat, the sympathetic nervous system is activated, prompting a release of cortisol and adrenaline, and the physiological preparation for 'fight or flight' (Evans 2019). The cognitive appraisal of stressors is subjective, 'If stressors actually do have a negative impact on individuals largely depends on appraisal and coping processes' (Lazarus and Folkman (1984), cited in Sonnentag and Fritz (2015, p. 74)). Midwives with less experience are more vulnerable to exaggerated cognitive appraisal, whereby a situation is perceived as unachievable due to a discrepancy in the complexity of care and capability of management, and therefore a potential threat to their well-being (Hearns 2022). In this situation, midwives are likely to use analytical cognitive processing, consciously considering the information and options available prior to decision making. This increases the cognitive load and is more time consuming. As the experience grows, the brain begins to look for patterns when approaching challenges, utilising automatic processing to address tasks. Automatic processing is quicker and less cognitively consuming (Kahneman 2013; Evans 2019).

So, how does the cognitive appraisal process link to behaviour? Whether a situation is perceived as a manageable challenge or a threat, both involve the release of

| Job Stressors | Examples | Reactions | Long term impact |
|---|---|---|---|
| Physical stressors (Extrinsic pressures) | Lack of resources (staff, equipment)<br>Working culture/environment<br>Shift work (night shifts)<br>Conflict in models of care (service needs vs. woman-centred care) | Acute/chronic<br><br>**Physical**<br>• Adrenaline surge<br>• Cortisol surge<br>• Increased HR<br>• Increased BP<br>• Increased RR<br>• Tense muscles<br>• Sweating<br>• Peripheral vision compromise<br>• Audible capacity decreases<br>• Poor sleep<br><br>**Psychological**<br>• Negative affect<br>• Stress<br>• Fatigue<br>• Anxiety<br>• Compassion fatigue<br>• Moral injury<br>• Difficulty decision-making<br>• Impaired long-term memory<br><br>**Behavioural:**<br>• Incivility<br>• Angry<br>• Withdrawn<br>• Miscommunication<br>• Defensive practice | • Exhaustion<br>• Burnout<br>• Poor health (e.g. cardiovascular disease)<br>• Absenteeism<br>• Poor job satisfaction<br><br>Mediators:<br>• Social support<br>• Leadership<br>• Psychological safety<br>• Coping mechanisms<br>• 'resilience'<br>• Reflection<br>• Self-efficacy<br>• Adaptability<br>• Clinical experience<br>• Disability<br>• Psychological detachment<br>• Proactive behaviours |
| Task-related stressors (Intrinsic pressures) | Time pressure<br>Work overload<br>Work complexity (clinical skill vs. experience)<br>Interruptions<br>Situational constraints<br>'With task' vs. 'with woman' | | |
| Role stressors | Role overload (acting up)<br>Role conflict (divided attention)<br>Role ambiguity<br>Supervision of junior staff and students | | |
| Social stressors | Unfamiliar team (pseudo team)<br>Incivility<br>Violence<br>Harassment<br>Abusive supervision<br>Bullying | | |
| Career-related stressors | Professional development opportunities<br>Continuous Professional Development (CPD) requirements<br>Work/life balance | | |
| Traumatic events | Obstetric & neonatal emergency<br>Neonatal/maternal death<br>Participating in poor care | | |
| Change processes | Policy & guideline updates<br>Equipment/technology<br>Trust/Maternity Service targets | | |

**Fig. 3.1**  Examples of job stressors, the bodily response and potential impacts

stress hormones. When a challenge is equitable to our skills, knowledge and resources, the hormones improve cognitive function and are productive in maintaining flow performance (Sandi 2013). If the challenge surmounts this, for example, with excessive pressure or cognitive load, the hormone response conditions the body in a state of defence, compromising physical and psychological capability. Whether the stressor is acute or chronic will modify the impact. Figure 3.1 gives examples of potential physical, psychological and behavioural reactions in response to work stressors identified by Sonnentag and Fritz (2015), including the long-term effects of these reactions (see Fig. 3.1).

When the midwives on a shift are largely junior or less experienced, the dynamic of the team changes. Considering the cognitive connotations of performance for inexperienced midwives, delegation of care needs to incorporate safety (Hearns 2022). This can increase the pressures and expectations of the experienced midwives within the team (see Sect. 3.6). Conversely, when shifts are short-staffed, this could increase the likelihood of a midwife being required to provide care that includes unfamiliar practice. If the pressure for any member of the team is considered too much, this results in cognitive overload and symptoms of stress. This can impact decision making, communication with the team and the ability to perform tasks requiring fine motor skills (Hearns 2022). For example, when responding to an obstetric haemorrhage emergency, if the team features less experienced midwives, the experienced midwife performing perineal repair may also be providing emergency management guidance to the inexperienced colleagues, thus dividing her attention and increasing the risk to safe task completion. Whilst a midwife's ability to assess pressure is individual, by creating awareness of the associated cognitive appraisal and by supporting management and handling through advanced and contemporaneous processes, performance is enhanced. This could include emergency proformas, structured format for assessment such as the foetal monitoring 'fresh care' review (National Institute for Health and Care Excellence 2022), risk assessment checklists and updated guidelines. Furthermore, similar to accepting and supporting the emotional burden that accompanies midwifery care, developing awareness of the detailed impact of intrinsic and extrinsic pressures midwives face can provide an informed advantage in addressing each pressure individually to achieve perceived control and a state of high-performance flow (Hearns 2022).

## 3.9    A Touch of Resilience

Although it remains a buzz word, resilience has lost its reputation as an advantageous trait and is fast becoming another way for the responsibility of a stress response to be placed with the individual rather than as a result of working conditions (Hunter and Warren 2022). Defined by Hunter and Warren (2014, p. 927) as the ability of an individual to respond positively and consistently to adversity, using effective coping strategies, research has highlighted the nature of the working environment as a moderator to sustainability and resilience in midwifery (Crowther et al. 2016).

When individual coping strategies are applied to adverse working conditions, does this promote resilience? Psychologist Jan Smith (2021) comments on concerns that the NHS is promoting staff to accept a system that is not fit for purpose through delivering resilience training, risking the potential for psychological harm:

> I hear those I support compare themselves to colleagues who appear unaffected, and the message they have received is they are struggling because they were not resilient enough, tough enough, thick-skinned enough. (Smith 2021, p. 104)

Greenstock (2023, p. 129) describes how it is:

> unspoken expectations, beliefs and obligations of the role as perceived by the employer and employee … the 'understood way of working' that in reality can be totally unacceptable but has become the norm. (Greenstock 2023, p. 129)

that can negatively impact resilience and self-awareness, demonstrating the contribution of the wider picture to the individual's perceived resilience.

The work by Dweck (2017) on the growth mindset discusses the potential for resilience and even achievement when facing challenges with a learning disposition. Dweck (2017) emphasises the importance of offering praise relating to the efforts of others irrespective of the outcome. This fosters the belief that performance is correlated to effort and approach, providing encouragement in the face of adversity. This is particularly significant in 'VUCA' working environments such as healthcare, where positive outcomes do not always result from measured strategy (Edmondson 2018).

Whilst more could be said regarding the individual resilience of midwives today, the focus should remain on the working environment. Despite its reputation faltering as a trait to possess, a number of organisational aspects have been identified that, when effectively modified, can promote a sense of resilience and sustainability amongst staff. This includes contribution to and control over working patterns, improved working conditions, quality role models and supervision allowing for openness and reframing of realities, reduced trauma exposure and structured support (Killian 2008; Croft 2022).

## 3.10 Midwife Skill and Experience

The time when resilience is perhaps most tested is at the beginning of a midwife's career. A lot of attention is paid to the early years of a midwife's career being the most vulnerable, with greater susceptibility to workplace stressors and subsequent negative impact to midwife well-being (Hunter and Warren 2014). Exploration into the resilience of newly qualified midwives has revealed that when a poor working culture is compounded by staffing issues and a lack of autonomy over working patterns, professional resilience is challenged (Bower 2023). In addition, being able to provide care that is safe and aligned with midwifery values, whilst having access to support as confidence and competence grows, develops professional affinity, which has the potential for reducing attrition (Capper et al. 2023). This chapter demonstrates the reality of the working environment and staffing issues in midwifery care represent multiple challenges for the newly registered midwives. This is particularly significant with the increase in pre-registration midwifery training places projecting a steady increase in newly qualified midwives (Health Education England 2019).

Where clinical experience is expected to increase competence and confidence with managing the ambiguity of maternity care, this is likely to expose midwives to women and birthing people of increasing complexity, and subsequently to potentially traumatic events. Therefore, increased experience does not protect from the potential psychological impacts of trauma (Mollart et al. 2013; Sheen et al. 2014). Staff with increased clinical experience are also often allocated multiple tasks or tasks that require 'acting up' within their role, increasing the cognitive load, which has the potential to delay acts of care (Hearns 2022). Whilst clinical skill and experience has the potential to act as a catalyst for a midwife's approach to some of the challenges identified, it is also important to consider the period of their career whereby knowledge and skill acquisition is perhaps at its most intense—during the 3-year midwifery degree. Student midwives are our future workforce; we are aware that some students leave their midwifery programmes and do not register as midwives when qualified (see Sect. 2.2), so understanding their experience of the midwifery working environment is essential.

## 3.11 Our Future Workforce

Midwifery is a popular course to study at undergraduate level, with a high number of applicants per place on midwifery degree programmes. However, student expectations and the reality of programmes can mean that some students drop out and do not complete their programmes. This has been made worse by the financial burden while completing programmes, as the NHS bursary was removed in 2017 and students rely on loans to pay their fees and living costs (Stacey 2024). The long hours on placements limit students' opportunities to undertake other paid work to support themselves (RCM 2024). Financial stresses have been implicated in the reduction of mature applicants onto healthcare programmes (Manthorpe and Baginsky 2023). Although the figures are not published for midwifery, 39% of undergraduate nursing students did not complete their programmes in UK universities in 2023 (Stacey 2024). Poor placements, workload and financial issues were the most common reasons for non-completion. Students reported being used to cover gaps in rotas and taking on support worker duties, over and above their opportunities for learning (Stacey 2024). The experience of student midwives on placement is outlined by McNeil and Kitson-Reynolds (2024). This work describes some positive experiences, but also some negative interactions such as: '*She completely looked past me and walked on, which I thought was really rude and it just made me think I don't want to work with this person* (p. 17). Another student worried about her future: *What kind of NHS are we going into? What kind of pressures are we going to have?...It's the workload and the conditions we will be working in, that's what put me off'* (p. 17).

The doctoral thesis entitled *The lived experiences of student midwives subjected to inappropriate behaviour* explores the impact of negative interactions.

> She did not directly ignore me, more that I was not overtly included in conversations or that her body was slightly turned away from me when she was speaking to others. The behaviours which I experienced were very subtle in nature and were difficult to articulate to others however, the impact of these subtle behaviours left me feeling inadequate. (Johnston 2016, p. 17)

Capper (2021) explored workplace bullying experienced by student midwives in both the UK and Australia in her thesis (Capper 2021). She describes student midwives leaving their programmes:

> Enthusiastic would-be midwifery students were applying to study midwifery in their droves, but once enrolled in their course, many lost their passion and enthusiasm and student numbers dwindled. (Capper 2021, p. 8)

The NHS Workforce Plan (NHS England 2023a) to recruit more student midwives may be insufficient to reassure organisations that the 'cavalry are coming' to shore up midwifery staffing levels. This is evident as some students choose not to join the profession even if they have completed and been successful in their degree. The environments for students and newly qualified staff are particularly worrying as described by Capper (2021) and Hawkins et al. (2019). Although students recognised the strain that staff were under, some noted that some *'cliques'* of midwives would help other members with their high workloads and leave others to struggle. One student said:

> I think midwives … are changed by the pressures and environment. Midwives are treated badly by their managers—this filters down to their treatment of students…—the lowest link in the chain. (Capper 2021, p. 177)

One concern is that students may be socialised into this behaviour and could replicate it themselves, further perpetuating the cycle. It is proposed the students own coping mechanisms could determine whether they are likely to replicate this behaviour (Hoel et al. 2007). If feelings are suppressed and students become 'hardened', they may see these experiences as normal events and be more likely to repeat them.

## 3.12   Enabling Students and Staff to Thrive

The Safe Learning Environment Charter was launched in February 2024 in response to learner's feedback on placements in maternity services and the need to develop positive learning cultures (NHS England 2024b). This is based on the experience of 2482 learners, educators and key stakeholders in health education in a bid to improve quality (Grimwood et al. 2023). Shortages in midwifery staffing were recognised; however, the need for time and space for learning was highlighted as a priority. The charter also calls for dedicated time for feedback to students, space for reflection and discussion of cases. The charter outlines *what good looks like,* stating that learners are to be respected and feel valued, and that staff should demonstrate good working relationships and civility. Zero tolerance to incivility, bullying and harassment is expected, together with the importance of role modelling NHS values (NHS England 2024b).

The Ockenden report calls for mechanisms to be in place to support the psychological and emotional needs of staff, in the recognition that well-supported teams are better able to deliver compassionate care (Ockenden 2022). This is a key feature of Schwartz Rounds (Point of Care 2015) and the role of the Professional Midwifery Advocates (PMAs) (Kerelo 2020). Schwartz Rounds provide the opportunity for students and staff to address their thoughts and feelings in response to the ethical, emotional, and social challenges of midwifery care (see Chap. 6). These rounds normalise caregiver emotions and are a welcome part of psychological safety in a positive workplace culture (Greenstock 2023).

Active Bystander training offers additional tools for managing workplace unprofessional behaviour. This training and simulation-based exercises have been shown to help medical students recognise and respond to disrespectful behaviour and could be considered for wider implementation (Aitken et al. 2023; Chew et al. 2023). Poor behaviour can be handled in the moment, but unless incidents are reported formally, there may be missed opportunities to identify patterns and address disrespectful and damaging behaviour in a timely way. Additionally, growing a culture of kindness has been developed into a Civility Toolkit for civility champions and PMAs to use (Capital Midwife and Health Education England 2021). This toolkit includes the Clark Workplace Civility Index, which can help broach conversations about civility in the workplace (Clark et al. 2018; Clark 2025). This work on civility relates to other initiatives such as the workforce behaviour toolkit developed jointly by the RCM and Royal College of Obstetricians and Gynaecologists (RCOG) (2021). Self-assess your own civility score by undertaking the Clark Workplace Civility Index assessment below; this is a valuable exercise made possible through the kind permission given by Dr Clark (Fig. 3.2).

Ask yourself, how often do I:
(5) almost always (4) usually (3) occasionally (2) rarely (1) almost never

1.Extend goodwill and think the best of others                                        1 2 3 4 5
2.Include and welcome new and current colleagues                                      1 2 3 4 5
3.Communicate respectfully (by e-mail, telephone, online, face-to-face)
   and really listen                                                                  1 2 3 4 5
4.Avoid spreading negative gossip and rumors                                          1 2 3 4 5
5.Keep confidences and respect others' privacy                                        1 2 3 4 5
6.Encourage, support, and mentor other staff                                          1 2 3 4 5
7.Avoid abusing my position or authority                                              1 2 3 4 5
8.Use respectful language (no racial, ethnic, sexual, gender, weight, age, ability,
   or religiously biased terms                                                        1 2 3 4 5
9.Attend meetings, arrive on time, participate, volunteer, and do my share            1 2 3 4 5
10.Avoid distracting others (misusing media, side conversations) during meetings.     1 2 3 4 5
11.Avoid taking credit for another individual's or team's contributions.              1 2 3 4 5
12.Acknowledge others and praise their work/contributions.                            1 2 3 4 5
13.Take personal responsibility and accountability for my actions                     1 2 3 4 5
14.Speak directly to the person with whom I have an issue                             1 2 3 4 5
15.Share pertinent or important information with others                               1 2 3 4 5
16.Uphold the vision, mission, and shared values of my organization.                  1 2 3 4 5
17.Seek and encourage constructive feedback from others.                              1 2 3 4 5
18.Demonstrate approachability, flexibility, and openness to other points of view     1 2 3 4 5
19.Bring my 'A' Game and a strong work ethic to my workplace.                         1 2 3 4 5
20.Apologize and mean it when the situation calls for it.                             1 2 3 4 5

Scoring the Workplace Civility Index: Add up the number of 1-5 responses to determine your own 'civility' score

90-100   Very civil
80-89    Civil
70-79    Moderately civil
60-69    Minimally civil
50-59    Uncivil

**My Total Civility Score =**

Fig. 3.2  Clark workplace civility index (Clark et al. 2018; Clark 2025). (The Clark Workplace Civility Index© is copyrighted material and may not be distributed or reproduced in any form without written permission from Dr. Cynthia Clark. A license to use the Clark Workplace Civility Index can be obtained by contacting techtransfer@boisestate.edu)

**Box 3.3 Exercise: How Civil Am I?**
Select the response that most accurately represents how true each statement to be. Enter the score for each item; then add the numbers to determine how civil you assess yourself to be. Scores range from 20 to 100.

## 3.13 Conclusions and Key Messages

In this chapter, we have learnt that the demand for midwifery care has changed, and care delivery has become more complex (NMC 2024). The midwifery workforce has become more junior and staffing pressures have intensified the workload. There is some evidence that increased pressure is linked with negative coping mechanisms if midwives go into survival or self-preservation mode. This may be a contributing factor to altered behaviour, affecting both themselves and the team around them (Fig. 3.3).

---

Midwifery understaffing is a global problem. Workload has increased due to the complexity in the population together with increased interventions.

Low staffing should not be normalised as it is associated with risks to families and to midwives themselves. Staffing levels that enable maternity staff to provide high quality care to women and neonates are essential.

When staffing is low, midwives prioritise safety over other key skills such as communication and teamwork

Low staffing may contribute to coping behaviours which are self-protective and may not be aligned to team cohesion.

The changing nature of midwifery work including shifts and pseudo teamworking, with the increasing complexity of the modern birthing person means midwives are needing to work progressively under pressure.

Retention of midwives is key to solving the workforce crisis however, some midwives feel disillusioned as they cannot provide the quality of care they would like to.

Midwives face a number of challenges in their role, including emotional labour of caring for families and unpredictable events. They may experience exhaustion, compassion fatigue and moral distress.

Rather than expressing frustration about staffing in a negative way, concerns should be escalated using organisation processes and external regulation if necessary.

Staffing is not an excuse for disrespectful behaviour, it is within midwives' power to retain professional standards and nurture other midwives, even in the face of heavy workloads.

A culture of psychological safety is identified as a 'golden thread of change' (OED 2025) and essential for effective team working and communication, encouraging transparency and candour, and promoting staff wellbeing.

A coping culture that prioritises the needs of the system, normalises poor working conditions, and prevents midwives from being 'with woman', can lead to moral injury and psychological ill-health.

Leadership, that encompasses compassion, vulnerability and humility, role models performance when under pressure and supports an inclusive learning culture for all.

A midwife's level of clinical experience impacts the cognitive processing of information and the management of workload, with professional resilience most susceptible for newly qualified midwives.

Negative interactions and unprofessional behaviour have been noted in periods of understaffing. Students and newly qualified staff are particularly vulnerable to the impact of this.

Psychological wellbeing has previously been the responsibility of the individual midwife, however recent literature has recognized the importance of a shared approach with systems and governing bodies, highlighting the necessity of a trauma-informed, supported midwifery workforce in ensuring high-quality, safe care.

Lack of support is contributing to midwifery students not completing their programmes or choosing not to join the professional register at the end of their studies, decreasing the future pipeline of midwives. The Safe Learning Environment Charter offers a quality standard for supporting learners.

---

**Fig. 3.3** Key messages

Workplace culture is multifaceted; the workload and pressure of the environment could have detrimental effects, especially in less robust teams. If disrespectful behaviour is tolerated and goes unchecked, this further diminishes confidence, teamwork and safety. A 'coping culture' avoids acknowledging and addressing midwives' psychological and physiological needs. However, by acknowledging the emotional aspect of midwifery care and establishing a systems approach to psychological staff well-being, this creates space for a trauma-informed midwifery workforce (Slade et al. 2018) that is accommodating of an individual's level of clinical experience and performance.

In the absence of a respectful, psychologically safe culture, the health of both the midwives and the families they care for is jeopardised. If the working conditions of midwives are not addressed and if the midwives themselves are not valued, this is likely to negatively affect the health and well-being of the perinatal population (World Health Organization (WHO) 2016). In concordance with the global review conducted by Carvajal et al. (2024), a practice environment that features proactive holistic support for midwives is integral to providing safe and respectful care for women and pregnant people. To begin to address midwife absenteeism and to create a respectful working environment, the psychological well-being of midwives needs to be valued, with a shared responsibility approach between individuals, teams, and organisational leaders (Maben et al. 2023).

# References


Aitken D, Shama H, Panchdhari A, Afonso de Barro S, Hodge G, Finch Z, George RE (2023) Twelve tips for developing active bystander intervention training for medical students. Med Teacher. 45(8):822–829

Adriaenssens J, De Gucht V, Maes S. Determinants and prevalence of burnout in emergency nurses: a systematic review of 25 years of research. Int J Nurs Stud. 2015;52(2):649–61.

Alexander C, Bogossian F, New K. Australian midwives and clinical investigation: Exploration of the personal and professional impact. Women Birth. 2021 ;34(1):38–47.

Aunger J, Maben J, Abrams R, Wright J, Mannion R, Pearson M, Jones A, Westbrook J (2023) Drivers of unprofessional behaviour between staff in acute care hospitals: a realist review. BMC Health Serv Res 23

Bimpong KA, Khan A, Slight R, Tolley C, Light SP (2019) Relationship between labour force satisfaction, wages and retention within the UK National Health Service: a systematic review of the literature. BMJ Open 10(7). https://doi.org/10.1136/bmjopen-2019-034919

Bloxsome D, Ireson D, Doleman G, Bayes S (2019) Factors associated with midwives' job satisfaction and intention to stay in the profession: An integrative review. Journal of clinical nursing 28(3–4): 386–399

Bogren M, Grahn M, Kaboru BB, Berg M (2020) Midwives challenges and factors that motivate them to remain in their workplace in the Democratic Republic of Congo – an interview study. Hum Resources Health. 18:1–10

Bonar S (2019) England short of almost 2,500 midwives, new birth figures confirm. Available at: https://www.rcm.org.uk/news-views/rcm-opinion/2019/england-short-of-almost-2-500-midwives-new-birth-figures-confirm

Bower H (2023) Resilience and retention in newly qualified midwives. European Journal of Midwifery. 7(Supplement 1). Available at https://doi.org/10.18332/ejm/172464

Brown B (2015) Daring greatly: How the courage to be vulnerable transforms the way we live, love, parent, and lead. Penguin Life, London

Capital Midwife and Health Education England (2021) Growing our culture of kindness: Civility Toolkit. Available at: https://www.hee.nhs.uk/sites/default/files/documents/CM%20civility%20toolkit%20March%2022.pdf

Capper T (2021) Workplace bullying: The midwifery student experience. Available at: https://acquire.cqu.edu.au/articles/thesis/Workplace_bullying_The_midwifery_student_experience/14776482/1/files/28395063.pdf

Capper TS, Haynes K, Williamson M (2023) How do new midwives' early workforce experiences influence their career plans? An integrative review of the literature. Nurse Education in Practice. 70(103689)

Care Quality Commission (2021) Regulation 18: Staffing. from https://www.cqc.org.uk/guidance-providers/regulations-enforcement/regulation-18-staffing (Accessed 28th April 2022)

Carvajal B, Hancock A, Lewney K, Hagan K, Jamieson S, Cooke A (2024) A global overview of midwives' working conditions: A rapid review of literature on positive practice environment. Women and Birth, 37:15–50

Catling C, Rossiter C (2020) Midwifery workplace culture in Australia: A national survey of midwives. Women and Birth 33:464–47

Chew C, Taylor E, Pope L, Nazir F, Paton C, Colquhoun K, Hunter I, Lydon E, Young D, O'Dwyer P (2023) Empowering future leaders: the value of simulation in active bystander training for medical students. BMJ Leader 7(S2)(S2)

Christoffersen L, Teigan J, Ronningstad C (2020) Following-up midwives after adverse incidents: How front-line management practices help second victims. Midwifery 85:102669

Chughtai AA, Buckley F (2013) Exploring the impact of trust on research scientists' work engagement. Personnel Review. 42(4):396–421

Civility Saves Lives (2024).Academic papers. Available at: https://www.civilitysaveslives.com/academic-papers

Clark C M, Sattler V, and Barbosa-Leiker C (2018) Development and psychometric testing of the Workplace Civility Index: A reliable tool to assess workplace civility, Journal of Continuing Education in Nursing, 49(9), 400–406

Clark CM (2025) Creating and sustaining civility in nursing education. 3rd ed. Sigma Theta Tau International Publishing

Cordey S, Moncrief G, Cull J, Sarian A, Powney D, Kindgon C, Feeley C, Downe S (2022) There's only so much you can be pushed: a commentary on the magnification of the maternity staffing crisis by the 2020/21 COVID-19 pandemic. British Journal of Obstetrics and Gynaecology 129:1408–1409

Coxon, K, Evans K, Thomson G, (2024) A response to the UK All Party Parliamentary Group report on Birth Trauma. Midwifery 137:104131

Coyle D (2018) The Culture Code: The Secrets of Highly Successful Groups. Random House, Manhattan

Creese J, Byrne JP, Conway E, O'Connor G, Humphries N (2024) They say they listen. But do they really listen?: A qualitative study of hospital doctors' experiences of organisational deafness, disconnect and denial. Health Services Management Research 0(0) 1–9

Croft E (2022) Factors affecting resilience: the role of ACEs, a coach-athlete relationship and shift-and persist. Undergraduate dissertation (unpublished)

Crown Prosecution (2011) Witness statement of Helene Donnelly: The Mid Staffordshire NHS Foundation Trust Public Inquiry. Available at: https://minhalexander.com/wp-content/uploads/2016/09/helen-donnelly-witness-statement-to-mid-staffs-public-inquiry.pdf

Crowther S, Hunter B, McAra-Couper J, Warren L, Gilkison A, Hunter M, Fielder A, Kirkham M (2016) Sustainability and resilience in midwifery: A discussion paper. Midwifery 40:40–48

Csikszentmihalyi M (1990) Flow: The psychology of optimal experience. Journal of Leisure Research, 24(1):93–94

Cull J, Hunter B, Henley J, Fenwick J, Sidebotham M (2020). Overwhelmed and out of my depth: Responses from early career midwives in the United Kingdom to the Work, Health and Emotional Lives of Midwives study. Women and Birth 33(6): e549–e557

Cummings GG, Tate K, Lee S, Wong CA, Paananen T, Micaroni SM, Chaterjee GE (2018) Leadership styles and outcome patterns for the nursing workforce and work environment: A systematic review. International Journal of Nursing Studies, 85, 9–60

Dall'Ora C, Meredith P, Saville C, Jones J, Griffiths P (2024). The association between nurse staffing configurations and sickness absence: longitudinal study. Available at: https://www.medrxiv.org/content/10.1101/2024.09.02.24312931v1

Darzi A (2024) Independent investigation of the National Health Service in England. Crown Copyright

Department of Health and Social Care (2024) Government issues rallying cry to the nation to help fix NHS. Available at: https://www.gov.uk/government/news/government-issues-rallying-cry-to-the-nation-to-help-fix-nhs [Accessed on 10 November 2024]

Dweck C (2017) Mindset: The New Psychology of Success. Penguin Random House: London

Edmondson AC (2018) The Fearless Organization: Creating Psychological Safety in the Workplace for Learning, Innovation, and Growth. Wiley: New Jersey

Evans C (2019) Perform under Pressure. Harper Collins Publishers: London

Feeley C, Stacey T (2024). Novel solutions to the midwifery retention crisis in England: an organisational case study of midwives' intentions to leave the profession and the role of retention midwives. Midwifery 104152: 104152

Ford M (2020) Midwives skipping meals and delaying toilet breaks, warns RCM. Nursing Times. Available at: Midwives skipping meals and delaying toilet breaks, warns RCM | Nursing Times [Accessed 7 October 2024]

Francis R (2013) Report of the Mid Staffordshire NHS Foundation Trust public inquiry: executive summary. 947, Available at: https://assets.publishing.service.gov.uk/government/uploads/system/uploads/attachment_data/file/279124/0947.pdf

Frese M, Keith N (2015) Action errors, error management, and learning in organisations. Annual Review of Psychology, 66(1):661–687

Gray S (2022) Sue Gray: Failure of leadership over Downing Street lockdown parties. Available at: https://www.bbc.co.uk/news/uk-politics-60203287 [Accessed on: 10 November 2024]

Geraghty S, Speelman C, Bayes S (2019) Fighting a losing battle: Midwives experiences of workplace stress. Women and Birth 32:297–306

Goleman D (2011) The brain and emotional intelligence: New insights. More Than Sound LLC: Northampton, MA

Greenstock K, (2023) Flourish. Printer and Martin Ltd, London

Grimwood T, Snell L, Hitchen S, Cotterell N, Ray S, Lake K (2023) Review of Midwifery Education and Training and Newly Qualified Experience: Thematic Analysis. Available at: https://www.england.nhs.uk/wp-content/uploads/2024/02/PRN00748i-review-of-midwifery-education-and-taining-and-newly-qualified-experience-thematic-analysis-haske-rep.pdf

Hawkins N, Jeong S, Smith T (2019) New graduate registered nurses' exposure to negative workplace behaviour in the acute care setting: An integrative review. International journal of nursing studies 93:41–54

Health Education England (2018) Reducing pre-registration attrition and improving retention report. Available at: https://www.hee.nhs.uk/sites/default/files/documents/RePAIR%20Report%202018_FINAL_0.pdf

Health Education England (2019) Maternity Workforce Strategy – Transforming the Maternity Workforce. Phase 1: Delivering the Five Year Forwards View for Maternity. Available at: https://www.hee.nhs.uk/sites/default/files/documents/MWS_ExecSummary_Web.pdf

Healy S, Humphreys E, Kennedy C (2016) Midwives' and Obstetricians' perceptions of risk and its impact on clinical practice and decision-making in labour: An integrative review. Women and Birth, 29(2):107–116

Hearns S (2022) Peak Performance Under Pressure: Lessons from a Helicopter Rescue Doctor. Class Professional Publishing, Somerset

Hoel H, Giga M, Davidson M (2007) Expectations and realities of student nurses' experiences of negative behaviour and bullying in clinical placement and the influences of socialization processes. Health Services Management Research 20:270–278

Hope J, Schoonhoven L, Griffiths P, Gould L, Bridges J. (2022). 'I'll put up with things for a long time before I need to call anybody': Face work, the Total Institution and the perpetuation of care inequalities. Sociology of health & illness 44(2): 469–487

Hunter B, Warren L (2014) Midwives' experiences of workplace resilience. Midwifery 30(8): 926–934

Hunter B, Warren L (2022) Revisiting Resilience. The Practicing Midwife 25: 9–13

James-Edwards D (2023) Unprofessional behaviours: actions need consequences. The Kings Fund Blog: Leadership and Workforce. Available at: https://www.kingsfund.org.uk/insight-and-analysis/blogs/unprofessional-behaviours-actions-need-consequences [Accessed on 10 November 2024]

Johnston J (2016) The lived experiences of student midwives subjected to inappropriate behaviour. Available at: https://eprints.soton.ac.uk/411282/1/Jane_Johnston_Thesis.pdf

Kahneman D (2013) Thinking fast and slow. New York, Farrar, Straus and Giroux

Kerelo S (2020) What is a professional midwifery advocate? British Journal of Midwifery 28(4):220–221

Killian KD (2008) Helping till it hurts? A multimethod study of compassion fatigue, burnout, and self-care in clinicians working with trauma survivors. Traumatology 24(2): 32–44

Kinman G, Teoh K, Harriss A (2020). The mental health and wellbeing of nurses and midwives in the United Kingdom. Available at: https://www.som.org.uk/sites/som.org.uk/files/The_Mental_Health_and_Wellbeing_of_Nurses_and_Midwives_in_the_United_Kingdom.pdf

Kirkup B (2015) The Report of the Morecambe Bay Investigation. Available at: http://data.parliament.uk/DepositedPapers/Files/DEP2015-0267/The_Report_of_the_Morecambe_Bay.pdf

Kivimaki M, Sutinen R, Elovainio M, Vahtera J, Räsänen K, Töyry S, Ferrie JE, Firth-Cozens J (2001) Sickness absence in hospital physicians: 2 year follow up study on determinants. Occupational and Environmental Medicine 58(6): 361–366

Lazarus RS, Folkman S (1984) Stress, appraisal and coping. Springer, New York

Love B, Sidebotham M, Fenwick J, Harvey S, Fairbrother G (2017) Unscrambling what is in your head: A mixed-method evaluation of clinical supervision for midwives. Women and Birth 30: 271–281

Maben J, Taylor C, Jagosh J, Carrieri D, Briscoe S, Klepacz N, Mattick K (2023) Delivering healthcare: a complex balancing act: A guide to understanding and tackling psychological ill-health in nurses, midwives and paramedics. University of Surrey, Guildford. www.workforceresearchsurrey.health

Manthorpe J, Baginsky M (2023) Midwives' morale, recruitment and retention–a rapid scoping review with some observations from the profession of social work. Available at: https://doi.org/10.18742/pub01-125

May DR, Gilson GL, Harter LM (2004) The psychological conditions of meaningfulness, safety and availability and the engagement of the human spirit at work. Journal of Occupational and Organizational Psychology 77(1):11–37

Mayra K, Catling C, Musa H, Hunter B, Bair K (2023) Compassion for midwives: The missing element in workplace culture for midwives globally. PLOS Global Public Health 3(7): e0002034

McCourt C, Olander E, Wiseman O, Uddin N, Plachcinski R, Rayment J, Lazar J, Ross-Davie M, Grollman C (2023) Independent evaluation of the implementation of midwifery continuity of carer. Available at: https://bpb-eu-w2.wpmucdn.com/blogs.city.ac.uk/dist/e/2879/files/2024/05/MCoC-evaluation-final-report-20.5.24.pdf

McNeil M, Kitson-Reynolds E (2024). Student midwives' experiences of clinical placement and the decision to enter the professional register. British Journal of Midwifery 32:14–20. Available: https://www.britishjournalofmidwifery.com/content/research/student-midwives-experiences-of-clinical-placement-and-the-decision-to-enter-the-professional-register/ (accessed 26 Jan 2025)

Mollart L, Skinner, VM, Newing C, Foureur M (2013) Factors that may influence midwives work-related stress and burnout. Women and Birth 26(1):26–32

Moncrieff G, Downe S, Maxwell M, Cheyne H (2023) Mapping factors that may influence attrition and retention of midwives: a scoping review protocol. BMJ open 13(10): e076686

National Guardian Office (2024) Culture is a patient safety issue: a summary of speaking up to freedom to speak up guardians 1 April 2023 – 31 March 2024. Available at: https://national-guardian.org.uk/wp-content/uploads/2024/07/FTSU-Case-Data-Annual-Report-23-24-1.pdf

National Institute for Health and Care Excellence (2022) NICE Guideline NG229: Fetal Monitoring in Labour. Available at: https://www.nice.org.uk/guidance/ng229/chapter/Recommendations [Accessed on: 1st October 2024]

Newnham E, Kirkham M (2019) Beyond autonomy: Care ethics for midwifery and the humanization of birth, Nursing Ethics, 26(708):2417–2157

NHS Digital (2023) Hospital Episode Statistics (HES). from https://digital.nhs.uk/data-and-information/publications/statistical/nhs-maternity-statistics/2022-23 (Accessed: 18th Jan 2024)

NHS England (2021) NHS Staff Survey Results: detailed spreadsheets. Available at: https://www.nhsstaffsurveys.com/results/results-archive/ [Accessed on: 1st October 2024]

NHS England (2023a). NHS long term workforce plan. Available at: https://www.england.nhs.uk/publication/nhs-long-term-workforce-plan/

NHS England (2023b) Staff Recognition Framework. Available at: https://www.england.nhs.uk/long-read/staff-recognition-framework/ [Accessed on 8th October 2024]

NHS England (2024a). Legacy mentoring. Available at: https://www.england.nhs.uk/looking-after-our-people/supporting-people-in-early-and-late-career/legacy-mentoring/

NHS England (2024b). Safe Learning Environment Charter. Available at: https://www.england.nhs.uk/mat-transformation/safe-learning-environment-charter/

Nove A, Friberg I, de Bernis L, McConville F, Moran A, Najjemba M, Ten Hoope-Bender, P, Tracy S, Homer CS (2021). Potential impact of midwives in preventing and reducing maternal and neonatal mortality and stillbirths: a Lives Saved Tool modelling study. The Lancet Global Health 9(1): e24–e32

Nursing and Midwifery Council (2019). The NMC register. T2019; (March):28. from https://www.nmc.org.uk/globalassets/sitedocuments/otherpublications/nmc-register-datamarch-19.pdf

Nursing and Midwifery Council (2020) Our Values and Behaviours. Available at: https://www.nmc.org.uk/about-us/our-role/our-values-and-mission/ [Accessed on 12th September 2024]

Nursing and Midwifery Council (2023) The NMC Register Mid-Year Update: 1st April – 30th September 2023. Available https://www.nmc.org.uk/globalassets/sitedocuments/data-reports/sep-2023/0130a-mid-year-data-report-uk-web.pdf (nmc.org.uk) [Accessed 8 October 2024]

Nursing and Midwifery Council (2024) Independent Culture Review. Available at: https://www.nmc.org.uk/globalassets/sitedocuments/independent-reviews/2024/nmc-independent-culture-review-july-2024.pdf [Accessed 12 September 2024]

Ockenden D (2022) Ockenden report – final: findings, conclusions and essential actions from the Independent Review of Maternity Services at The Shrewsbury and Telford Hospital NHS Trust. (HC1219). Available https://assets.publishing.service.gov.uk/media/624332fe8fa8f527744f0615/Final-Ockenden-Report-web-accessible.pdf [Accessed 10 November 2024]

Oxford English Dictionary (2025) Oxford University Press. Oxford Available at: https://www.oxfordlearnersdictionaries.com/definition/english/golden-thread?q=golden+thread (Accessed 28 Feb 2025)

Peyman A, Nayeri ND, Bandboni ME, Moghadam ZB (2017) The experience of litigation from the perspective of midwives in Iran. J. Forensic Nurs 13(135)

Rathert C, Ishqaidef G, May DR (2009) Improving work environments in healthcare: test of a theoretical framework. Healthcare Management Review 34(4); 334–343

Reed A (2020) Overdue: Birth, burnout and a blueprint for a better NHS. Pinter and Martin Ltd, London

Renfrew MJ, McFadden AMH, Bastos MH, Campbell J, Channon AA, Cheung NF, Silva DRAD, Downe S, Kennedy HP, Malata A (2014) Midwifery and quality care: findings from a new evidence-informed framework for maternal and newborn care. The Lancet 384(9948): 1129–1145

Robertson JH, Thomson AM (2016) An exploration of the effects of clinical negligence litigation on midwives in England: a phenomenological study. Midwifery 33: 55–63

Sandi C (2013) Stress and Cognition. Wiley Interdisciplinary Reviews: Cognitive Science 4(3): 245–261

Royal College of Midwives (2022a) RCM Survey of Midwives and MSWs in England. Available at: https://pre.rcm.org.uk/rcm-survey-of-midwives-and-msws-in-england/ (Accessed on, 1 October 2024

Royal College of Midwives (2022b) RCM evidence to the NHS Pay Review Body. Available at: https://www.rcm.org.uk/media/5784/rcm-pay-review-body-evidence-2022.pdf#:~:text=The%20Royal%20College%20of%20Midwives%20%28RCM%29%20welcomes%20the,and%20maternity%20support%20workers%20%28MSWs%29%20in%20the%20UK

Royal College of Midwives (2024) State of UK midwifery student finance. Available at: https://rcm.org.uk/wp-content/uploads/2024/09/rcm_state-of-uk-midwifery-student-finance-report.pdf

Royal College of Nursing (2024) NHS Staff Survey shows nursing and midwifery staff facing almost every type of abuse. Available at: https://www.rcn.org.uk/news-and-events/Press-Releases/nhs-staff-survey-shows-nursing-and-midwifery-staff-facing-almost-every-type-of-abuse

Royal College of Obstetricians and Gynaecologists (2021) RCOG and RCM joint statement on undermining and bullying in the workplace. Available at: https://www.rcog.org.uk/careers-and-training/starting-your-og-career/workforce/improving-workplace-behaviours/rcog-and-rcm-joint-statement-on-undermining-and-bullying-in-the-workplace/

Rydon-Grange M (2018) Psychological perspective on compassion in modern healthcare settings. J Med Ethics 44(11): 729–733

Schmiedhofer M, Derksen C, Keller FM, Dietl JE, Häussler F, Strametz R, Koester-Steinebach I, Lippke S (2021) Barriers and facilitators of safe communication in obstetrics: results from qualitative interviews with physicians, midwives and nurses. International journal of environmental research and public health 18(3): 915

Sheen K, Slade P, Spiby H (2014) An integrative review of the impact of indirect trauma exposure in health professionals and potential issues of salience for midwives. Journal of Advanced Nursing 70(4): 729–743

Sheen K, Spiby H, Slade P (2016) The experience and impact of traumatic perinatal event experiences in midwives: A qualitative investigation. International Journal of Nursing Studies 53:1–72

Slade P, Sheen K, Collinge S, Butters J, Spiby H (2018) A programme for the prevention of post-traumatic stress disorder in midwifery (POPPY): indications of effectiveness from a feasibility study. European Journal of Psychotraumatology 9(1)

Smith J (2021) Nurturing Maternity Staff. Pinter and Martin, London

Sonnentag S, Fritz C (2015) Recovery from job stress: The stressor-detachment model as an integrative framework. Journal of Organizational Behaviour 36: 72–103

Spence SM (2023) I'm just a number, I'm not a person, I'm just a servant to the system: introducing a new conceptual framework to understand bullying in NHS midwifery. Doctoral dissertation. University of Leeds

Spencer L (2015) Rise and Shine: Recover from burnout and get back to your best. Rethink Press: Norfolk

Stacey A (2024) Nursing students: why are almost 40% leaving before they qualify? https://rcni.com/nursing-standard/newsroom/analysis/nursing-students-why-are-almost-40-leaving-they-qualify-208246

Stockdale M (2023) Seeing both sides: wellbeing in maternity services post COVID-19. Available at: https://research.bangor.ac.uk/portal/files/59885598/2023_Stockdale_MJ_DClinPsy.pdf

Taylor B, Cross-Sudworth F, Rimmer M, Quinn L, Morris RK, Johnston T, Morad S, Davidson L, Kenyon S, UK Audit Research Collaborative in Obstetrics Gynaecology Members (2024)

Induction of labour care in the UK: A cross-sectional survey of maternity units. PLoS One 19(2): e0297857

Taylor C, Mattick K, Carrieri D, Cox J, Maben J (2022) 'The WOW factors': comparing workforce organization and well-being for doctors, nurses, midwives and paramedics in England. British medical bulletin 141(1): 60–79

The Point of Care Foundation (2015) Schwartz Rounds. Available: http://www.pointofcarefoundation.org.uk/our-work/Schwartz-rounds/ (accessed 4 Feb 2025)

Turner L (2021) Evidence base on case load held practice and outcomes, in E. Kitson-Reynolds and K. Ashforth (Eds) (2021) A Concise Guide to Continuity of Care in Midwifery. Routledge: 34–52

Turner L, Ball J, Meredith P, Kitson-Reynolds E, Griffiths P (2024) The association between midwifery staffing and reported harmful incidents: a cross-sectional analysis of routinely collected data. BMC Health Serv Res 24: 1–8

West M (2012) Effective Teamwork: Practical lessons from organizational research. Third edition. Blackwell Publishing, Oxford

West M (2021) Compassionate Leadership: Sustaining Wisdom, Humanity and Presence in Health and Social Care. The Swirling Leaf Press, London

World Health Organization (2016) Midwives' voices, midwives' realities. Findings from a global consultation on providing quality midwifery care. World Health Organization: Geneva

Wyeman J (2024) Pressure on maternity services show no sign of lessening. Available at: https://www.wrighthassall.co.uk/knowledge-base/pressure-on-maternity-services-show-no-sign-of-lessening [Accessed on 7th October 2024]

# The Future of Midwifery Rests with Our Students: Can You Meet the Challenge?

**4**

Ellen Kitson-Reynolds and Marie Naish

## 4.1 Introduction

While written primarily for student midwives, this chapter can be helpful for newly qualified midwives, practice supervisors and assessors, practice education teams and midwifery educators. This chapter is about illuminating what is within each person for them to find and develop from. Domain 5 in the Nursing and Midwifery Council (NMC) standards of proficiency for midwives (NMC 2019) states that at the point of qualification and entry to the register, graduates must:

> 5.14 demonstrate how to recognise signs of vulnerability in themselves or their colleagues and the actions required to minimise risks to health or wellbeing of self and others.
> 5.15 demonstrate awareness of the need to manage the personal and emotional challenges of work and workload, uncertainty, and change; and incorporate compassionate self-care into their personal and professional life. (NMC 2019)

Upon completion of your pre-registration midwifery education in the United Kingdom (UK), you will have attended a minimum of 2300 h in clinical practice, amounting to 50% of your pre-registration training. During this time, you will have seen the best of the profession, care provision and service delivery, leaving you to celebrate the reasons you chose midwifery as a career. You will have also experienced clinical situations, which have challenged you to the core, leading you to question why you chose midwifery as your career. This is the reality of midwifery practice, both as a student and moving forward through your chosen career (Kitson-Reynolds 2010).

E. Kitson-Reynolds (✉) · M. Naish
University of Southampton, Southampton, United Kingdom
e-mail: E.L.Kitson-Reynolds@soton.ac.uk; M.E.Naish@soton.ac.uk



M. O'Brien, E. Kitson-Reynolds (eds.), *Respectful Relationships in the Maternity Service*, https://doi.org/10.1007/978-3-032-04281-1_4

This chapter explores how pre-registration education informs, challenges and enhances the impact of the student journey on preparing you for contemporary midwifery in practice. We consider what compassion, empathy and emotional intelligence are and how they promote a compassionate and kind culture within midwifery practice. We present a values-based curriculum lens and consider how it could improve the experiences of students through their education. Throughout this chapter, we will pause to ask you to apply concepts to your real-world experiences of midwifery education and for you to forward project how this could impact your future career, care provision and how you will support future learners in both your student role and as a qualified midwife.

## 4.2    What Does Midwifery Mean to Me?

Choosing a career in midwifery is often influenced by a motivation to care (Wareing et al. 2024), achieved by entering a profession that offers a rewarding opportunity to make a difference to the care of women and their families (Bloxsome et al. 2020). Despite this, according to Oates et al.'s (2020) descriptive qualitative study, student midwives in England described their experiences as a 'rollercoaster' with multiple culture shocks whilst continually moving between university and numerous clinical placements. The midwifery pre-registration training programme is a constant period of change. It is stated that the training programme is an extreme test of the students' emotional resilience while being balanced by times of elation (Oates et al. 2020). It will be of no surprise to you reading this that students in Oates et al.'s (2020) study described their training as 'relentless' with no opportunity for breaks to look after oneself in the practice setting.

When considering the NMC (2019) standard 5.15, as outlined at the start of this chapter, self-care could include requiring one to take breaks and identify when changes and workloads start to become overwhelming, without just walking away from the shift allocation or the profession altogether. Oates et al. (2020) conclude that developing confidence is important to helping students cope with midwifery education programme challenges, which include developing their professional interactions with healthcare professionals in clinical environments. If you can resonate with these findings, and if the challenge is overwhelming, you may have started to question why you are still following this career trajectory. Before you continue with this chapter, it would be helpful if you complete Exercise 4.1 below.

**Box 4.1 Exercise: The Fairy Tale of Midwifery Versus the Reality of the Role**
When we embark on a new adventure, we have created in our mind what we envisage the journey will entail.

1. Spend some time recalling your utopic vision of what you thought the role of the midwife is and why you decided midwifery was the career for you.
2. Think about a typical day in practice, how does this day differ from what you thought the role of a midwife is, or how does this day meet your expectations?
3. How did the difference in your expectations, values and beliefs linked to the role of the midwife affect the way in which you behave in practice?
4. What is it about midwifery that keeps you getting out of bed in the morning to carry on doing the role?

Based on Kitson-Reynolds (2010) and Kitson-Reynolds et al. (2014)

This activity requires you to be honest with yourself, which may leave you feeling vulnerable (Brown 2015). We all have days where we shout, 'Yes! This is why I am doing this!' and which remind you why you chose to undertake your midwifery education and at this time in your life. You are experiencing first-hand the reality of the clinical care provision and the positive impact you are having with those you encounter. You are learning about you, how you think, function and what drives you to achieve for yourself and provide best care for women and their families; all the time, you are role modelling for the next generations of students. This may leave you feeling vulnerable and, at times, exhausted. Brown (2015) asserts that through this vulnerability, we learn and become stronger. You are the future of the midwifery profession, and it is a positive reminder to you that you have the strength to achieve.

## 4.3   Compassion, Empathy and Emotional Intelligence Promote a Compassionate and Kind Culture Within Midwifery Practice

Compassionate culture is a phrase you may have heard a great deal of in recent times within the media (Wei 2023), health-related policy and reports (National Health Service England, [NHSE] n.d.; Alderwick and Dunn 2024), standards of proficiency for midwives (NMC 2019) and a plethora of academic publications. So, what is compassion and why does it appear prolific? It is not a new concept as Gu et al. (2017) suggest; however, it has a growing interest in psychology as being part of 'humanness'. Compassion has roots in spirituality, primarily in Buddhist psychology and within three concepts: self-kindness, mindfulness and a sense of common humanity (Harrison 2022). One can enhance this thinking by adding humility as a related concept. Cultural humility is filtering through contemporary healthcare to better support compassionate healthcare (So et al. 2024; Tsuchida et al. 2023). Buddhist traditions refer to duality, meaning self and others; hence, compassion brings about social connectedness (Barker et al. 2023), promoting respectful (NHS Values 2024) and positive cultures that are more likely to be altruistic in nature (Weiss-Sidi and Riemer 2023). Guo et al. (2019) assert that prosocial behaviour promotes harmonious relationships intended to benefit others, identifying a link to people being more honest, having greater intelligence, exhibiting values in fairness, justice, social responsibility and individuals identifying as a 'moral' person. Understanding individual personality traits may also impact these behaviours, although this has not yet been factored into the research discussions.

Studies (Soosalu et al. 2019; Dunn et al. 2010; Klara et al. 2014; Aziz and Thompson 1998) postulate that humans have three 'brains' that process numerous stimuli around them. These three 'brains' interlink and are the head, heart and gut. Each of these systems deals with the impact, effect and actions individuals take when positioned in certain circumstances. Each system has its own neurons that process and interpret the environment, people, emotion and body language around us. Typically, our intuitive responses take into consideration not only our personality traits but how compassionate, kind and fatigued we presently feel. Each of the three 'brains' guides how we respond and what dialogue we instinctively use. The head supports the consciousness, the language we use and cognition (Perlovsky and Ilin 2012). The heart deals with emotions (Dunn et al. 2010), expression of values and the interpersonal connections and the gut controls self-preservation (Klara et al. 2014; Aziz and Thompson 1998) and how we cope with challenges, which may include poor workplace cultures. Barnes et al. (2010) studied differences between the male and female brain, identifying through MRI scanning that the female corpus callosum is thicker than the male, insinuating that women experience greater intuition and processing of feelings. This is perhaps unsurprising, as many of us would accept that from experience females tend to feel and express emotion more freely than their male counterparts; however, this may be a social construct (Lively 2024). Males are not always prompted to express emotion from childhood, which may or may not link to cultural upbringing (Di Bianca and Mahalik 2022) and observed differences between men and women.

Compassionate healthcare impacts whether patients live or die (Watts et al. 2023; Turner et al. 2024a) and alleviates work-related burnout and compassion fatigue (Beaumont et al. 2016; Hansel and Saltzman 2023; Todaro-Franceschi 2024; Dall'ora et al. 2020). It is well documented that the current maternity workforce is burnt out and has compassion fatigue (Garnett et al. 2023; Todaro-Franceschi 2024), which manifests through the numbers of midwives leaving the profession within 5 years of qualifying if, indeed, they do decide to enter the professional register at the point of qualification (Royal College Midwives [RCM] (2016). As such, the RCM (2023), NHS and NMC have woken up to the fact that attrition rates remain high, resulting in proactive actions such as the Reducing Pre-registration Attrition and Improving Retention (RePAIR) report (NHSE 2018), explicit pre-registration standards for midwifery within Domain 5 (NMC 2019) and the NHS workforce plan (NHSE 2023). Compassion is one of six core NHS values outlined in the NHS Constitution (Department of Health and Social Care [DHSC] 2023). Compassionate healthcare is identified as being integral, not only because it captures the humanness of care and is the correct approach to take for patient satisfaction but also because a compassionate culture within healthcare services is directly linked to safety and improved outcomes (DHSC 2023). There are significant consequences when kindness and compassion are lacking; please take some time to consider Activity 4.2.

---

**Box 4.2 Exercise: What Does Compassion Mean to Me?**
Please reflect on a compassionate clinical experience:
Describe the situation and your involvement.

How did you feel?
How did the other people involved respond to the compassionate experience?
What is the key learning point for you to take into your future practice?

Reflect on an uncompassionate clinical experience:
Describe the situation and your involvement.

How did you feel?
How did the other people involved respond to the uncompassionate experience?
What is the key learning point for you to take into your future practice?
How do the two experiences compare?

What are the key points from this reflection that you will take to your future practice?

---

Many texts refer to the need for kindness, tolerance and compassion in all areas of society (Michel et al. 2024). For staff to provide compassionate care, it is important that they feel valued and supported, for example, there has been a focus within retail linked television advertisements reminding the public that their employees deserve and expect kindness. These messages are explicit such as the Co-operative group stating that they expect customers to show kindness to their shop staff through upholding their core values 'owned by you, right by you' to '.... stop the abuse of shop workers....' (Co-op 2024). The NHS has been asserting this expectation for several years with messaging such as 'zero tolerance' (Gabe and Elston 2008; Bennett 2001; Merivale 2020).

Lord Darzi was commissioned to review the state of the NHS in 2024 by the newly elected Labour government Darzi (DHSC 2024); he concludes that the NHS is in a critical condition as a combined result of a lack of capital investment during a period of high demand and deteriorating national health. While the road to recovery is likely long, Darzi (DHSC 2024) draws on the importance of re-engaging staff who, despite low morale and significant service challenges, continue to show their commitment to improving the quality of care.

Whilst this review has been welcomed by many, there are critics who have highlighted what the Darzi (DHSC 2024) report has omitted (Kline 2024; Alderwick and Dunn 2024). It is worth noting that maternity services barely received a mention, stating that *'capacity for compassion is variable, sensitive to environment and pressure, but can be systematically improved'* (DHSC 2024), with the RCM releasing a response:

> While some areas of the NHS will be praising this report and its findings, capacity remains a major concern among our members. The midwifery community wants to provide the best quality, safest care to women and families but they can't do that if they are having to fight for crumbs from the table. (RCM 2024)

Workplace culture (see Sect. 2.7.3) has resulted in staff disengagement, high sickness rates, bullying, discrimination, poor staff well-being, failure to value, support and develop staff (Singh et al. 2023). These environments lead to compassion fatigue, which in turn leads to inability to demonstrate emotional intelligence (Garnett et al. 2023). These 'toxic behaviours' are considered to have normalised poor behaviours in the NHS (Averbuch et al. 2021).

It is reported that *civility saves lives* (Silver-MacMahon 2023). NHS human factors training includes reminding professional groups of the impact kindness has on patient care (Pierce et al. 2023). Incivility has the potential to impact effective teamworking, with Pierce et al.'s (2023) study demonstrating the effect of poor workplace behaviours on inter-professional relationships, in this study, impeding the effective management of obstetric emergencies. Consequently, Kline (2024) emphasises the need to have kindness at all levels regardless of roles and positions. Pre-registration education includes reviewing workplace cultures and its impact on safe patient care. If students do not see kindness and compassion in clinical placement, as has been documented by Arundell et al. (2018), it would be understandable as to why they may not believe what they are taught in higher education institutions about successful working environments. Patients watch the behaviours in practice with students concerned that the perception on patient care is poor (Capper et al. 2021a, b). Gu et al. (2017) refer to Strauss et al.'s (2016) review of 'existing conceptualisation' of what compassion comprises, defining the five elements of compassion.

The five elements of compassion (Strauss et al. 2016) are as follows:

1. Recognising suffering
2. Understanding the universality of suffering in human experience
3. Feeling moved by the person suffering and emotionally connecting with their distress
4. Tolerating uncomfortable feelings aroused so that we remain open to and accepting of the person suffering
5. Acting or being motivated to act to alleviate suffering

Gu et al. (2017) challenge the fourth concept of 'tolerating' as being 'problematic' and 'not a core element of compassion'. However, one can consider this further in clinical practice by asking if clinicians do 'tolerate' feeling uncomfortable to immerse oneself into the experiences of others or, if due to a perceived lack of time or workloads, if it is easier to omit this to be able to juggle the competing demands in allocated work time. If one considers self-compassion, it may provide a sense of psychological safety to remove such an emotional construct to be able to achieve something to the best of one's ability. Gu et al. (2017) suggest that this does not detract from being compassionate, as it can better support being compassionate to others, but to the detriment of self. It could be that our personalities sub-consciously guide us to wanting to pursue a career in health and caring for others, whilst failing to care for ourselves. If time is a compounding factor to achieving step 4, perhaps as clinicians, we should consider what we should and are prepared to tolerate. To consider this fully, one needs to consider the plethora of activity linked to workloads and staffing (see Chap. 3).

Di Lorenzo et al.'s (2019) research concluded that nursing students' emotional competence is essential for professional practice. Emotional competence comprises empathy and emotional intelligence. Pre-registration education and clinical experience support the development of skills used to recognise and understand how another person feels, how best to support their wishes, how to act as their advocate and how to 'communicate…' these emotions '…*effectively and with kindness and compassion…*' (NMC 2019) to those who may be involved in inter-professional care provision (Igbokwe et al. 2023). Emotional intelligence is the means to recognise and manage one's own emotions (Harahap et al. 2023) whilst having the skill to influence another's emotions (Drigas et al. 2023). Emotional intelligence is linked with empathy; however, it has been suggested that empathy and interpersonal competence have largely been ignored in favour of technological advances and knowledge (Terry and Cain 2016). Perhaps unsurprisingly, Di Lorenzo et al.'s (2019) research concludes that nurses, and, by association, midwives need skills in emotional intelligence to better understand their patients' perspectives and have a high level of empathy. Evidence suggests that those with higher emotional intelligence are more likely to be leaders in their field (Harahap et al. 2023), have effective critical thinking skills (Sk and Halder 2024) and generally have better therapeutic relationships (Chung et al. 2023). Emotional intelligence and compassion are inextricably linked by alleviating suffering and extending kindness (Strauss et al. 2016; Wood 2024; Huber 2023) and so have the foundations in building positive cultures and healthy professional and personal relationships (Walker and Wright 2024).

Domain 5 (NMC 2019) encourages student midwives to develop self-care. Through self-compassion and a strength-based approach come greater resilience and greater professional satisfaction (Di Lorenzo et al. 2019), better mental health and less negative stress (Coldridge and Davies 2017; Martínez-Rubio et al. 2023). Self-compassion is to be able to be compassionate to others (Heffernan et al. 2010). Beaumont et al.'s (2016) purposive quantitative survey, with a sample of 103 university educated student midwives, found that just over half of students exhibited high levels of burnout, while students who showed self-compassion had less compassion fatigue and burnout than those who were deemed to be harsh or less forgiving on themselves. This had a direct impact on the student's mental well-being, and how much compassion students gave to others. There is a range of support available, with students encouraged to seek support via a Professional Midwifery Advocate (PMA) (Kerelo 2020), receive trauma risk management (TRiM) support (Long et al. 2024) and access freedom to speak out guardians (Delpino et al. 2023), line managers (Clarkson et al. 2023), practice assessors or supervisors and academic assessors (NMC 2023). It is hoped that students who experience positive support are more likely to have confidence to challenge poor behaviours and provide support and guidance to future learners, colleagues and women and birthing people in the moment.

## 4.4    A Values-Based Curriculum to Enhance the Experiences of Students Through Their Education

It is acknowledged that there is a need to train and educate healthcare professionals to be kind and compassionate (NMC 2019) and thus live and breathe values that espouse professional behaviours and expectations. The world appears to be more complex since the global pandemic in 2020. The cost of living has impacted most households, not just those from lower socio-economic status, causing instability (Douglas 2024; Calafati et al. 2023) and insecurity from continuous change and challenges to well-being in all areas of life (Di Fabio and Saklofske 2021; Michel et al. 2024). Psychology texts point to a need for strength-based interventions (Silverman et al. 2023; Park 2020; Gupta et al. 2021), which the NMC are capitalising on (NMC 2019) in a bid to address current workforce issues (Turner et al. 2024b). With advances in technology and artificial intelligence (AI) coming to healthcare, increasing patient and health worker demands and expectations (Garnett et al. 2023), normalisation of life post-COVID, the want to have a healthy workplace, perhaps therefore, there is a need to be showing more compassion and core values (NHS Core Values 2024; Michel et al. 2024). AI provides the machine learning, but cannot apply the emotions or emotional interpretations. Training in cultivating compassion ultimately enhances compassion (Slavich et al. 2022). There is a recognition of the need to enhance the understanding of equality, diversity, inclusivity and belonging (EDIB) throughout the curriculum (RCM 2023) to improve outcomes for women and birthing people and neonates from Black, Asian and Mixed Ethnic groups and those living in deprivation, while also supporting the retention and progression of staff within the NHS through improved experience and workplace culture (RCM 2023). Kitson-Reynolds and Ashforth (2022) highlight professional values linked to continuity of care throughout their 'Autism friendly' curriculum, including ensuring that all students and academics undertake active bystander training (Robertson and Steele 2023), complete a values-based enquiry (VBE) journey (Kitson-Reynolds 2020, 2022) and undertake academic modules written to espouse kindness and compassion.

As described by Kitson-Reynolds and Ashforth (2022, p. 162), the University of Southampton 'Bachelor of Science (HONS) Midwifery' programme has a strong values-based ethos to learning to enable [students] to demonstrate caring through evidence of a commitment to valuing each person for whom [they] care'. Students undertake activities to reflect on their personal values and belief systems to better understand themselves, develop resilience and/or a strength-based approach (Saleebey 2013), demonstrate graduate attributes (Oraison et al. 2019) and value inter-professional education and team working in clinical practice to enhance care provision and health outcomes for those they encounter in practice settings. Having this level of emotional intelligence promotes confidence in an increased ability to understand, control and manage their own emotions (Heffernan et al. 2010). Hence, the values-based journey espoused a number of key NHS and NMC documents including local NHS Trust values statements, *Compassion in Practice* (Commissioning Board Chief Nursing Officer and DH Chief Nursing Adviser 2012), *Leading Change Adding Value'* (see Fig. 4.1) (NHS England 2016), *The Lancet Series* (Renfrew et al. 2014), *Strengthening Quality Midwifery Education* (World Health Organisation [WHO] 2019), *Standards for pre-registration midwifery programmes* (NMC 2019) and the 6 Cs (Cummings and Bennett 2012). Students are timetabled for eight sessions throughout the academic year in the theory weeks, each session being 3 h in length, facilitating time for both a personal academic tutor interaction and the VBE planned activity.

The VBE planned activities span the full duration of the programme, in this case, 3 years. There is a spiral development whereby the students expand their knowledge and explore their 'selves' alongside, reflecting on their personal values and beliefs and those they come into contact with, both in clinical practice (both women and

| Commitment No | Leading Change Adding Value Commitment |
|---|---|
| 1 | We willpromotea culture where improving thepopulation's healthis a core component of the practice of all nursing, midwifery and care staff |
| 2 | We will increase the visibility of nursing and midwifery leadership and input in prevention |
| 3 | We will work with individuals, families and communities to equip them to make informed choices and manage their own health |
| 4 | We will be centred on individuals experiencing high value care |
| 5 | We will work in partnership with individuals, their families, carers and others important to them |
| 6 | We will actively respond to what matters most to our staff and colleagues |
| 7 | We will lead and drive research to evidence the impact of what we do |
| 8 | We will have the right education, training and development to enhance our skills, knowledge and understanding |
| 9 | We will have the right staff in the right places and at the right time |
| 10 | We will champion the use of technology and informatics to improve practice, address unwarranted variations and enhance outcomes |

**Fig. 4.1** The 10 commitments of leading change

birthing people and clinical colleagues). The humanised philosophy is paramount and a constant throughout the curriculum design and delivery. By being so, the activities embrace societal and university core values and are linked to the ten commitments (NHS England 2016) as shown in Fig. 4.1. Students explore learning disabilities, self-awareness, communication, cultural competence, human rights, recycling and sustainability. The sessions utilise a seminar structure, encouraging students to reflect alone or in groups, have class-wide discussions and debates or quietly contemplate the 'you' as an individual. The aim is for the student to challenge themselves and others to think and devise their own plan for becoming the midwife they set out to be, and possibly more than they hoped for. By knowing the 'you' better, the hope is to become a stronger and more resilient practitioner for the future. Anecdotally, the VBE journey has shown positive development of emotional intelligence throughout the 3 years on programme, which mirrors the findings in Di Lorenzo et al.'s (2019) study. From experience, students embark on their journey to 'becoming a midwife' (Kitson-Reynolds 2010; Kitson-Reynolds et al. 2014) as passionate individuals wanting to give their all to those they provide care to, acting as advocates for the families in their care. This passion, linked with their personal values and belief systems, can at times be conflicting to the reality they experience, but with better self-understanding can develop their inner strength, cognitive and emotional intelligence, which, as Chavez Alvarez (2023) states, can lead to profound acts of kindness.

Students and qualified colleagues reflect the experiences they encounter in practice. Students often seek guidance from educators when they witness poor behaviours in clinical and educational environments. Students have a fresh perspective of what is right and wrong when it impacts clinical environments and vulnerable women and birthing people. They raise concerns and meet to debrief and develop the skills to challenge what they see throughout their education to improve the culture and, in turn, care outcomes. From our experiences, students are the powerful voices behind change, often calling upon organisations to see the impact of their actions on others. It leads one to question: why are they the perceived few, the strongest voice with the courage to stand up? Our experience is that the woman's voice is what drives the newer generations to provide best care and perhaps, you/they can see it, have the fresh eyes to it and are the less jaded in healthcare settings.

Midwifery is a global profession (Renfrew and Malata 2021). Health services serve a culturally diverse population (Heffernan et al. 2010). Service users and clinical colleagues from a wide range of cultural backgrounds and heritages support and shape an inclusive service design and delivery to better meet the needs of those accessing care. Midwifery education providers embrace international students to widen perspectives and understanding of worldviews. This rich, diverse culture supports learners and educators to embrace difference, be inclusive and to meet the global profession expectations. There is a greater acceptance and tolerance of difference in society (Hjerm et al. 2020); whilst education includes greater awareness of

EDIB for the women and birthing people that students provide care for and interact with, more healthcare professionals enter their professions equally with EDIB needs. Although admission practices are becoming more inclusive, the reality in practice is that culture in some universities and maternity units needs to change to be more inclusive of Black and Asian students. Recent reviews of maternity services have identified racism (Kirkup 2022; CQQ 2024), which does impact Black and Asian student midwife experience (see Sects. 2.4 and 8.3.2). The 'Autism friendly' curriculum considers neurodiverse needs for self, students, clinical colleagues, other clinicians and service users. As Di Lorenzo et al. (2019) inform, alexithymia is the condition where an individual cannot feel or express verbally their emotions; so, then, how does one navigate the clinical world with or without reasonable adjustments to safely provide care and meet the requirements of the professional code (NMC 2019)? If, as Heffernan et al. (2010) assert, emotions are important in relationships and communication with everyone who encounters health services either as service users or care providers, students are required to develop compassion and empathy skills, which can be achieved through the VBE journey.

Over recent years, it has been recorded that there is increasing dissatisfaction in aspects of nursing care in the NHS (Francis 2013) and, specifically, maternity services (Independent Maternity Review 2022; Kirkup 2015, 2022). Complaints include lack of courtesy (Baker and Brookes 2021), poor listening skills, not being able to explain things in a way that service users comprehend and not showing kindness (van Dael et al. 2020). Social media is a recent tool that surfaces poor practices and behaviours in many areas of life, organisations and society. Messaging is instant. It is out there in the wider world within seconds; that which may have once been hidden is available for all to see and is a powerful force to manage. Some of this has truth and others that may not be as truthful (Aïmeur et al. 2023) or appropriate to share. Rowse (2023) suggests that with the expansion of social media, now, more than ever, people need to develop their intuition to navigate new non-physical predators. Trusting one's intuition indicates when we feel dread, inspired, noticing patterns in our daily routines, which result in the sub-conscious and conscious reactions akin to fight or flight or carry on as typical. The environments in which students engage with, and how they cope with these, will therefore have an impact on their ability to develop and provide kind and compassionate care to patients. The VBE journey aims to equip students with skills to become compassionate individuals (Kitson-Reynolds 2020) who take pride in what they undertake; are grateful; show and have commitment; are pro-social (Guo et al. 2019); help others; and live for positive outcomes (Di Fabio and Saklofske 2021). The challenge for the future is how to refresh and update the VBEs to meet the new demands of societal changes and expectations of both individuals as future healthcare professionals and those to whom midwifery care is offered.

## 4.5 The Student Experience of Being 'Valued' Through the Lens of Pre-registration Student Midwives' Research Project

Midwifery students at the University of Southampton undertake a final-year project related to any aspect of midwifery practice including service evaluation, non-NHS research or an evidence-based project. Students undergo University ethics for service evaluation and research projects. McNeil and Kitson-Reynolds (2024) undertook a small non-NHS qualitative research project using interpretive phenomenological analysis (IPA) following principles of Smith et al. (2022). The purpose was to understand if student midwives were likely to leave their programme of education because of their experiences in clinical practice placements, thus having impact upon increasing a future qualified workforce. Student midwives within England were approached via a social media post and a total of student midwives who met the criteria were invited to attend semi-structured interviews. Seventy-nine themes were categorised into two super-ordinate themes: 'kindness and compassion grow future midwives and strength' and 'resolve through COVID-19 and beyond'. The overarching theme from the participants' interviews was 'I can be a good midwife when I qualify'. Key findings include the basic need to look at the individual student and the level of knowledge and experience they hold to determine the amount of support that is required, thus following a similar approach to individualised care planning for the service users. All students want to feel like they will be good midwives. This can be achieved through the positive role modelling from clinical colleagues towards the students throughout their clinical placements. Clinical colleagues from all professions who provide care to women birthing people and newborns should ensure that they show students civility and patience while teaching and supporting them. Students do not appreciate feeling belittled in front of those they were providing care to, as they feel undermined and not trusted to carry out the basic activities expected of them. This small research project confirms the concerns that many involved in the delivery of education hear on a regular basis and often recall experiencing ourselves as students.

The future of the midwifery profession depends on you to support and nurture the future workforce. You may already be undertaking aspects of this role as a senior student. Reflect on your own experiences and find out whether you are up for the challenge by completing the SWOT (Swann et al. 2022; Nichol et al. 2024) analysis in Activity 4.3.

**Box 4.3 Activity: 'Me' as the Future Practice Supervisor**

1. Undertake a SWOT (Swann et al. 2022; Nichol et al. 2024) analysis to reflect upon your experiences of learning and being supported by the practice supervisors and practice assessors you have encountered so far in your education.

| Strengths | Limitations or weaknesses |
|---|---|
| Opportunities | Threats |

2. Consider the points that you dislike about your experiences. How can you turn these into something positive in terms of your development and future practices as a student and/or qualified midwife?
3. Now, consider what type of supervisor you see yourself as, using a SWOT analysis (Swann et al. 2022; Nichol et al. 2024).

| Strengths | Limitations or weaknesses |
|---|---|
| Opportunities | Threats |

4. Is there anything within your SWOT that you would like to change about yourself and or develop further?

1. Write a personal development plan using SMART(ER) objectives (Swann et al. 2022; Nichol et al. 2024) that you can take into your future career.

| Specific | Measurable | Achievable | Realistic | Timed | Evaluated | Revised |
|---|---|---|---|---|---|---|
|  |  |  |  |  |  |  |

2. How compassionate do you think you are currently and what do you measure this against?
3. How compassionate will you be with your supervisee and how will you know if you are delivering to this belief?
4. When considering these questions, do you/how much do you consider your personal life experiences?
5. How much do you live up to the expectations you place on yourself and how do you know when these are not as you wish?
6. Whom do you reach out to for honest feedback and how do you hear the messages that you may or may not want to receive?

## 4.6    Conclusion

This chapter has explored varied experiences of pre-registration midwifery students. The essential principles of compassion, empathy and emotional intelligence have been discussed, including their influence on the safety of maternity care. Next, it has been considered how these attributes promote kind, compassionate cultures within maternity services. One approach to developing these attributes for student midwives has been described, the value-based education journey. The future of the midwifery profession *does* rest with you. Are you up for this challenge?

## References

Aïmeur E, Amri S, Brassard G (2023) Fake news, disinformation and misinformation in social media: a review. Social Network Analysis and Mining, 13(1): p. 30.

Alderwick H, Dunn P (2024) Darzi's NHS review shows depth of problems for Labour. BMJ 386. Available: https://doi.org/10.1136/bmj.q2032 (Accessed 24 Feb 2025)

Arundell F, Mannix J, Sheehan A et al (2018) Workplace culture and the practice experience of midwifery students: A meta-synthesis. J Nurs Manag 26(3):302–313. Available: https://doi.org/10.1111/jonm.12548 (Accessed 24 Feb 2025)

Averbuch T, Eliya Y, Van Spall HGC (2021) Systematic review of academic bullying in medical settings: dynamics and consequences. BMJ Open 11(7). Available: https://doi.org/10.1136/bmjopen-2020-043256 (Accessed 24 Feb 2025)

Aziz Q, Thompson DG (1998). Brain-gut axis in health and disease. Gastroenterology. 114(3) pp. 559–578.

Baker P, Brookes G (2021) Lovely nurses, rude receptionists, and patronising doctors Determining the impact of gender stereotyping on patient feedback. In The Routledge Handbook of Language, Gender, and Sexuality (pp. 559–571). Routledge.

Barker ME, Leach KT, Levett-Jones T (2023) Patient's views of empathic and compassionate healthcare interactions: a scoping review. Nurse Education Today 131. Available: https://doi.org/10.1016/j.nedt.2023.105957 (Accessed 24 Feb 2025)

Barnes J, Ridgway GR, Bartlett J et al (2010) Head size, age and gender adjustment in MRI studies: a necessary nuisance? NeuroImage 53(4):1244–1255. Available: https://doi.org/10.1016/j.neuroimage.2010.06.025 (Accessed 24 Feb 2025)

Beaumont E, Durkin M, Martin CJH et al (2016) Compassion for others, self-compassion, quality of life and mental well-being measures and their association with compassion fatigue and burnout in student midwives: A quantitative survey. Midwifery 34:239–244. Available: https://doi.org/10.1016/j.midw.2015.11.002 (Accessed 24 Feb 2025)

Bennett S (2001). Tackling violence in the NHS. BMJ, 323 (Suppl S2).

Bloxsome D, Bayes S, Ireson D (2020) "I love being a midwife; it's who I am": A Glaserian Grounded Theory Study of why midwives stay in midwifery. J Clin Nurs 29(1–2):208–220. https://doi.org/10.1111/jocn.15078

Brown B (2015) Rising Strong. Vermillion, London

Calafati L, Froud J, Haslam C, Johal S, Williams K (2023) When nothing works: from cost of living to foundational liveability. Manchester University Press, Manchester

Capper TS, Muurlink OT, Williamson MJ (2021a) The parents are watching: Midwifery students' perceptions of how workplace bullying impacts mothers and babies. Midwifery 103. Available: https://doi.org/10.1016/j.midw.2021.103144 (Accessed 24 Feb 2025)

Capper TS, Muurlink OT, Williamson MJ (2021b) Social culture and the bullying of midwifery students whilst on clinical placement: A qualitative descriptive exploration. Nurse Education in Practice 52. Available: https://doi.org/10.1016/j.nepr.2021.103045 (Accessed 24 Feb 2025)

Chavez Alvarez S. (2023) Kindness is the highest form of intelligence. Available at: https://medium.com/@projectmanagementandleadership/kindness-is-the-highest-form-of-intelligence-90a951cf244c#:~:text=Passion%20drives%20us%20to%20channel,kindness%20for%20those%20around%20us (Accessed 30 Dec 2024)

Chung SR, Cichocki MN, Chung KC (2023). Building emotional intelligence. Plastic and Reconstructive Surgery, 151(1), pp. 1–5.

Clarkson C, Scott HR, Hegarty S, et al (2023) 'You get looked at like you're failing': A reflexive thematic analysis of experiences of mental health and wellbeing support for NHS staff. Journal of Health Psychology 28(9):818–831. Available: https://doi.org/10.1177/13591053221140255 (Accessed 24 Feb 2025)

Coldridge L, Davies S (2017) "Am I too emotional for this job?" An exploration of student midwives' experiences of coping with traumatic events in the labour ward. Midwifery 45:1–6. Available: https://doi.org/10.1016/j.midw.2016.11.008 (Accessed 24 Feb 2025)

Commissioning Board Chief Nursing Officer and DH Chief Nursing Adviser (2012) Compassion in Practice. Leeds, Department of Health

Co-op (2024) Owned by you right by you, TV Advertisement. Available: https://www.youtube.com/watch?v=pva5UfbfZ9o&t=2s (Accessed 30 Dec 2024)

Cummings J, Bennett V (2012) Compassion in Practice: Nursing, Midwifery and care staff our vision and strategy. Department of Health, Leeds.

Care Quality Commission (2024) National Review of Maternity Service 2022 – 2024. Available: https://www.cqc.org.uk/publications/maternity-services-2022-2024 (Accessed 5 Feb 2025)

Dall'ora C, Ball J, Reinius M et al (2020) Burnout in nursing: A theoretical review. Human Resources for Health 18(41). Available: https://doi.org/10.1186/s12960-020-00469-9 (Accessed 24 Feb 2025)

Department of Health and Social Care. Independent investigation of the NHS in England. (2024). Available: https://www.gov.uk/government/publications/independent-investigation-of-the-nhs-in-england (Accessed 24 Feb 2025)

Delpino R, Lees-Deutsch L, Solanki B (2023) 'Speaking Up' for patient safety and staff wellbeing: a qualitative study. BMJ Open Quality, 12.

Department of Health and Social Care (2023) NHS Constitution. Available: https://www.gov.uk/government/publications/the-nhs-constitution-for-england/the-nhs-constitution-for-england#nhs-values (Accessed 25 Feb 2025).

Di Bianca M, Mahalik JR (2022). A relational-cultural framework for promoting healthy masculinities. American Psychologist, 77(3), p. 321.

Di Fabio A, Saklofske DH (2021) The relationship of compassion and self-compassion with personality and emotional intelligence. Pers Individ Dif. 2021 Feb 1;169:110109. Epub 2020 May 11. PMID: 32394994; PMCID: PMC7211602. Available: https://doi.org/10.1016/j.paid.2020.110109 (Accessed 24 Feb 2025)

Di Lorenzo R, Venturelli G, Spiga G, Ferri P (2019) Emotional intelligence, empathy and alexithymia: a cross-sectional survey on emotional competence in a group of nursing students. Acta Biomed. 2019 Mar 28;90(4-S):32–43. https://doi.org/10.23750/abm.v90i4-S.8273. PMID: 30977747; PMCID: PMC6625563. Available: https://pubmed.ncbi.nlm.nih.gov/30977747/ (Accessed 24 Feb 2025)

Douglas F (2024) What qualitative research can tell us about food and nutrition security in the UK and why we should pay attention to what it is telling us. Proceedings of the Nutrition Society, 83(3): pp. 170–179.

Drigas A, Papoutsi C, Skianis C (2023). Being an Emotionally Intelligent Leader through the Nine-Layer Model of Emotional Intelligence—The Supporting Role of New Technologies. Sustainability, 15(10): p. 8103.

Dunn B, Galton H, Morgan R, Evans D, Oliver C, Meyer M, Cusack R, Lawrence AD, Dalgleish T (2010) Listening to your heart: How interoception shapes emotion experience and intuitive decision making. Psychological Science 21(12):1835–1844. Available: https://doi.org/10.1177/0956797610389191 (Accessed 24 Feb 2025)

Francis R (2013) Report of the Mid Staffordshire NHS Foundation Trust public inquiry: executive summary [online] The Stationary Office. Available: https://assets.publishing.service.gov.uk/government/uploads/system/uploads/attachment_data/file/279124/0947.pdf (Accessed 26 Jan 2025)

Gabe J, Elston AM (2008). 'We don't have to take this': Zero tolerance of violence against health care workers in a time of insecurity. Social Policy & Administration, 42(6), pp. 691–709. Available            https://onlinelibrary.wiley.com/doi/abs/10.1111/j.1467-9515.2008.00632.x (Accessed 24 Feb 2025)

Garnett A, Hui L, Oleynikov C et al (2023) Compassion fatigue in healthcare providers: a scoping review. BMC Health Services Research 23:1336. Available: https://doi.org/10.1186/s12913-023-10356-3 (Accessed 24 Feb 2025)

Gu J, Cavanagh K, Baer R, Strauss C. An empirical examination of the factor structure of compassion. PLoS One. 2017 Feb 17;12(2): e0172471. https://doi.org/10.1371/journal.pone.0172471. PMID: 28212391; PMCID: PMC5315311.

Gupta A, Jagzape A, Kumar M, (2021). Social media effects among freshman medical students during COVID-19 lock-down: An online mixed research. Journal of Education and Health Promotion, 10(1): p. 55. Available: https://doi.org/10.4103/jehp.jehp_749_20 (Accessed 24 Feb 2025)

Guo Q, Sun P, Cai M, Zhang X, Song K (2019) Why are smarter individuals more prosocial? A study on the mediating roles of empathy and moral identity. Intelligence 75:1–8. Available: https://doi.org/10.1016/j.intell.2019.02.006 (Accessed 24 Feb 2025)

Hansel TC, Saltzman LY (2023) Secondary traumatic stress and burnout: The role of mental health, work experience, loneliness and other trauma in compassion fatigue in the healthcare workforces. Traumatology 30(4):615–618. Available: https://doi.org/10.1037/trm0000478 (Accessed 24 Feb 2025)

Harahap MAK, Sutrisno S, Mahendika D, Suherlan S, Ausat AMA (2023).The Role of Emotional Intelligence in Effective Leadership: A Review of Contemporary Research. Al-Buhuts, 19(1): pp. 354–369.

Harrison S (2022) What does self-compassion really mean. Available: https://hbr.org/2022/12/what-does-self-compassion-really-mean (Accessed 29 Oct 2024)

Heffernan M, Quinn Griffin MT, McNulty SR, Fitzpatrick JJ (2010). Self-compassion and emotional intelligence in nurses. Int J Nurs Pract 16(4):366–73. Available: https://doi.org/10.1111/j.1440-172X.2010.01853.x (Accessed 24 Feb 2025)

Hjerm M, Eger MA, Bohman A et al (2020) A new approach to the study of tolerance: Conceptualizing and measuring acceptance, respect, and appreciation of difference. Social Indicators Research 147(3):897–919. https://doi.org/10.1007/s11205-019-02176-y

Huber, D.H., 2023. Using a Self-Compassion Intervention to Increase Undergraduates' Emotional Intelligence (Doctoral dissertation, Idaho State University).

Igbokwe IC, Egboka PN, Thompson CC, Etele AV, Anyanwu AN, Okeke-James NJ, Uzoekwe HE (2023). Emotional intelligence: practices to manage and develop it. European Journal of Theoretical and Applied Sciences, 1(4): pp. 42–48.

Independent Maternity Review (2022) Ockenden report – Final: Findings, conclusions, and essential actions from the independent review of maternity services at the Shrewsbury and Telford Hospital NHS Trust (HC 1219) Crown. Available at https://assets.publishing.service.gov.uk/government/uploads/system/uploads/attachment_data/file/1064302/Final-Ockenden-Report-web-accessible.pdf (Accessed 9th Sept 2024)

Kerelo S (2020) What is a professional midwifery advocate? British Journal of Midwifery 28(4):220–221.

Kirkup B (2022) Reading the signals, Maternity and Neonatal Services East Kent – the report of the independent investigation. London: His Majesty's Stationary Office. Available: https://assets.publishing.service.gov.uk/media/634fb083e90e0731a5423408/reading-the-signals-maternity-and-neonatal-services-in-east-kent_the-report-of-the-independent-investigation_print-ready.pdf (Accessed 28 Jan 2025)

Kirkup B (2015). The Report of the Morecambe Bay Investigation. Preston: Morecambe Bay Investigation Copyright.

Kitson-Reynolds E (2010). The Lived Experience of Newly Qualified Midwives. Thesis, University of Southampton, UK Available: https://eprints.soton.ac.uk/193561/ (Accessed 24 Feb 2025)

Kitson-Reynolds and Ashforth (2022) Ch10: Resources In E. Kitson-Reynolds, and K. Ashforth, (Eds) A Concise Guide to Continuity of Care in Midwifery (pp. 149–175) London and New York: Routledge

Kitson-Reynolds E (2020) The University of Southampton Midwifery Values Based Enquiry Journey. University of Southampton: Southampton

Kitson-Reynolds (2022) Chapter 1, Introduction. In Kitson-Reynolds E and Ashforth K, (Eds) A Concise Guide to Continuity of Care in Midwifery (pp. 18–33) Routledge, London and New York:

Kitson-Reynolds E, Cluett E, Le-May A (2014) Fairy tale midwifery—fact or fiction: The lived experiences of newly qualified midwives. British Journal of Midwifery 22(9):660–668.

Klara M, Arnold M, Gunther L, Winter C, Langhans W, Meyer U (2014). Gut vagal afferents differentially modulate innate anxiety and learned fear. Journal of Neuroscience. 34: 7067–7076.

Kline, R (2024) What Darzi missed out, HSJ. Available: https://www.hsj.co.uk/workforce/what-darzi-missed-out/7037851.article (Accessed 10 Oct 2024)

Lively KJ (2024). Theories of Emotions. In Scarantino A (Ed) Sociology. Emotion Theory: The Routledge Comprehensive Guide: Volume I: History, Contemporary Theories, and Key Elements. Routledge, UK

Long T, Aggar C, Grace S (2024) Trauma-informed care education for midwives: Does education improve attitudes towards trauma-informed care? Midwifery 131. Available: https://doi.org/10.1016/j.midw.2024.103950 (Accessed 24 Feb 2024)

Martínez-Rubio D, Colomer-Carbonell A, Sanabria-Mazo JP et al (2023) How mindfulness, self-compassion, and experiential avoidance are related to perceived stress in a sample of university students. Plos One 18(2). Available: https://doi.org/10.1371/journal.pone.0280791 (Accessed 24 Feb 2025)

McNeil M, Kitson-Reynolds E (2024) Student midwives' experiences of clinical placement and the decision to enter the professional register. British Journal of Midwifery 32:14–20. Available: https://www.britishjournalofmidwifery.com/content/research/student-midwives-experiences-of-clinical-placement-and-the-decision-to-enter-the-professional-register/ (Accessed 26 Jan 2025)

Merivale J (2020). Violent and aggressive patients. BDJ Team, 7(7): pp. 24–25.

Michel J, Pham-Tan O, Tanner M (2024). Kindness leadership needed now more than ever, in global health and beyond? Journal of Global Health, 14.

NHS England (2016) 'Leading Change Adding Value' NHS England, Leeds

NHS Values (2024) The NHS Values. Available: https://www.healthcareers.nhs.uk/working-health/working-nhs/nhs-constitution (Accessed 24 Feb 2025)

NHS England (ND) (n.d.) We are compassionate and inclusive. Available: https://www.england.nhs.uk/looking-after-our-people/the-programme-and-resources/we-are-compassionate-and-inclusive/ (Accessed 24 Feb 2025)

NHS England (2023) The long-term workforce plan. Available: https://www.england.nhs.uk/long-read/nhs-long-term-workforce-plan-2/ (Accessed 24 Feb 2025)

NHS England (2018) RePAIR report. Available: https://www.hee.nhs.uk/our-work/reducing-pre-registration-attrition-improving-retention (Accessed 24 Feb 2025)

Nichol B, Kemp E, Wilson R et al (2024) Establishing an updated consensus on the conceptual and operational definitions of Making Every Contact Count (MECC) across experts within research and practice: an international Delphi Study. Public Health, 230:29–37. Available: https://doi.org/10.1016/j.puhe.2024.01.023 (Accessed 24 Feb 2025)

Nursing and Midwifery Council (2019) Standards for Pre-registration Midwifery Programmes. Nursing and Midwifery Council, London. Available: https://www.nmc.org.uk/globalassets/sitedocuments/standards/2024/standards-of-proficiency-for-midwives.pdf (Accessed 24 Feb 2025)

Nursing and Midwifery Council (2023) Standards for student supervision and assessment. Nursing and Midwifery Council, London.

Oates J, Topping A, Watts K, Charles P, Hunter C (2020) 'The rollercoaster': A qualitative study of midwifery students' experiences affecting their mental wellbeing. Midwifery 88. Available: https://doi.org/10.1016/j.midw.2020.102735 (Accessed 24 Feb 2025)

Oraison H, Konjarski L, Howe S (2019) Does university prepare students for employment? Alignment between graduate attributes, accreditation requirements and industry employability criteria. Journal of Teaching and Learning for Graduate Employability, 10(1): pp. 173–194.

Park RJ (2020) Mindfulness-Based Strengths Practice: A 'Toolbox' for Self-Efficacy in Higher Education (Doctoral dissertation, University of Lincoln).

Pierce H, Bone J, Carlisle E, Darcy M, Grant L, Verma G, Kermack A (2023) Demonstrating the impact of incivility in an obstetric emergency: An interventional simulation study. Authorea Preprints.

Perlovsky L and Ilin R, (2012). Brain. Conscious and unconscious mechanisms of cognition, emotions, and language. Brain Sciences, 2(4): pp. 790–834.

Renfrew MJ, Malata AM (2021) Scaling up care by midwives must now be a global priority. The Lancet Global Health 9(1):e2–e3. https://doi.org/10.1016/S2214-109X(20)30478-2

Renfrew MJ, McFadden A, Bastos MH et al (2014) Midwifery and quality care: findings from a new evidence-informed framework for maternal and newborn care. The Lancet 384(9948):1129–1145. https://doi.org/10.1016/S0140-6736(14)60789-3

Robertson A, Steele S (2023). A cross-sectional survey of English NHS Trusts on their uptake and provision of active bystander training including to address sexual harassment. JRSM open, 14(4), p. 20542704231166619.

Rowse J, (2023) No filter: technology-facilitated sexual assault of children and adults. Medical Journal of Australia. 218(11): pp. 506–508.

RCM (2023) England: State of maternity services 2023 London, RCM. Available: https://www.pslhub.org/learn/patient-safety-in-health-and-care/high-risk-areas/maternity/state-of-maternity-services-report-england-rcm-12-july-2023-r9855/ (Accessed 24 Feb 2025)

Royal College Midwives (2016) Why midwives leave – revisited. RCM, London. Available: https://cdn.ps.emap.com/wp-content/uploads/sites/3/2016/10/Why-Midwives-Leave (Accessed 24 Feb 2025)

RCM (2024) RCM responds to Darzi report Available: https://rcm.org.uk/media-releases/2024/09/rcm-responds-to-darzi-report/#:~:text=While%20some%20areas%20of%20the,for%20crumbs%20from%20the%20table.%E2%80%9D (Accessed 13 Jan 2025)

Saleebey D (Ed.) (2013). The strengths perspective in social work practice (6th ed.). Allyn and Bacon, Boston, MA

Silver-MacMahon H (2023). Civility saves lives: explaining why behaviour matters. In Practice 45(9): pp. 567–571. Available: https://doi.org/10.1002/inpr.374 (Accessed 24 Feb 2025)

Silverman DM, Rosario RJ, Hernandez IA, Destin M. The Ongoing Development of Strength-Based Approaches to People Who Hold Systemically Marginalized Identities. Pers Soc Psychol Rev. 2023 Aug;27(3):255–271. https://doi.org/10.1177/10888683221145243. Epub 2023 Jan 12. PMID: 36632745. Available: https://pubmed.ncbi.nlm.nih.gov/36632745/ (Accessed 24 Feb 2025)

Singh S, Meghrajani I, Vijh G, Thomas JP, Mohite S (2023). Relationship between workplace incivility, employee performance and employee engagement in healthcare institutions. Asia Pacific Journal of Health Management, 18(2): pp. 251–260.

Sk S, Halder S (2024). Effect of emotional intelligence and critical thinking disposition on resilience of the student in transition to higher education phase. Journal of College Student Retention: Research, Theory & Practice, 25(4): pp. 913–939. Available: https://journals.sagepub.com/doi/abs/10.1177/15210251211037996 (Accessed 24 Feb 2025)

Slavich GM, Roos LG, Zaki J (2022). Social belonging, compassion, and kindness: Key ingredients for fostering resilience, recovery, and growth from the COVID-19 pandemic. Anxiety, Stress, & Coping, 35(1): pp. 1–8.

Smith JA, Flowers P, Larkin, M (2022). Interpretive Phenomenological Analysis (2nd ed) Sage Publications

So N, Price K, O'Mara P, Rodrigues M A (2024) The importance of cultural humility and cultural safety in health care. The Medical Journal of Australia 220(1):12–13. Available: https://doi.org/10.5694/mja2.52182 (Accessed 24 Feb 2025).

Soosalu G, Henwood S, Deo A (2019). Head, heart, and gut in decision making: Development of a multiple brain preference questionnaire. Sage Open. 9(1): p. 2158244019837439.

Strauss C, Lever Taylor B, Gu J, Kuyken W, Baer R, Jones F, Cavanagh K. What is compassion and how can we measure it? A review of definitions and measures. Clin Psychol Rev. 2016 Jul;47:15–27. https://doi.org/10.1016/j.cpr.2016.05.004. Epub 2016 May 26. PMID: 27267346. Available: https://pubmed.ncbi.nlm.nih.gov/27267346/ (Accessed 24 Feb 2025)

Swann C, Jackman P C, Lawrence A, Hawkins, RM, Goddard S G, Williamson O, Ekkekakis P (2022). The (over)use of SMART goals for physical activity promotion: A narrative review and critique. Health Psychology Review, 17(2),211–226. Available: https://pubmed.ncbi.nlm.nih.gov/35094640/ (Accessed 21 Sept 2025)

Terry C, Cain J (2016). The emerging issue of digital empathy. American journal of pharmaceutical education, 80(4): p. 58.

Todaro-Franceschi V (2024). Compassion fatigue and burnout in nursing: Enhancing professional quality of life. Springer Publishing Company, London

Tsuchida RE, Doan J, Losman ED, Haggins AN, Huang RD, Hekman DJ, Perry MA (2023). Cultural humility curriculum to address healthcare disparities for emergency medicine residents. Western Journal of Emergency Medicine, 24(2), p. 119.

Turner L, Ball J, Meredith P et al (2024a) The association between midwifery staffing and reported harmful incidents: a cross-sectional analysis of routinely collected data. BMC Health Services Research 24(391). https://doi.org/10.1186/s12913-024-10812-8

Turner LY, Saville C, Ball J et al (2024b) Inpatient midwifery staffing levels and postpartum readmissions: a retrospective multicentre longitudinal study. BMJ Open 14(4). https://doi.org/10.1136/bmjopen-2023-077710

Van Dael J, Reader TW, Gillespie A et al (2020) Learning from complaints in healthcare: a realist review of academic literature, policy evidence and front-line insights. BMJ Quality & Safety 29(8):684–695. https://doi.org/10.1136/bmjqs-2019-009704

Wareing M, Newberry-Baker R, Sharples A, Pye S (2024) Career motivation of 1st year nursing and midwifery students: A cross-sectional study. International Journal of Practice-based Learning in Health and Social Care 12(1):115–126. Available: https://doi.org/10.18552/ijpbl-hsc.v12i1.966 (Accessed 24 Feb 2025)

Walker MS, Wright L (2024). A Historical and Empirical Review of Compassion. International Journal for Human Caring, 28(1).

Watts E, Patel H, Kostov A, Kim J, Elkbuli A (2023). The role of compassionate care in medicine: toward improving patients' quality of care and satisfaction. Journal of Surgical Research, 289, pp. 1–7.

Wei J (2023). Kindness in British communities: Discursive practices of promoting kindness during the Covid pandemic. Discourse & Society, 34(4): pp. 502–520. Available: https://pmc.ncbi.nlm.nih.gov/articles/PMC9834622/ (Accessed 24 Feb 2025)

Weiss-Sidi M, Riemer H (2023). Help others—be happy? The effect of altruistic behavior on happiness across cultures. Frontiers in psychology, 14, p. 1156661.

WHO (2019) Strengthening quality midwifery education for universal health coverage 2030: Framework for Action. WHO, Geneva

Wood J (2024). The Kindness Fix: How and Why, We Must Build a More Compassionate Society. Policy Press.

# Coaching: The 'Golden Thread of Change'

**5**

Denise Linay and Helen Rogers

## 5.1 Introduction

> Coaching is about enabling individuals to make conscious decisions and empowering them to become leaders in their own lives. (Wise 2020)

This chapter reinforces how the promotion and use of coaching are not only a key element of cultural change but can be transformational when a genuine coaching mind set is an established practice for all employees. This chapter explores how coaching can be a powerful tool for those who want to achieve a strong, supportive culture. It dispels the assumption that coaching is just for senior leaders; instead, it shows how not just formal coaching but also a coaching approach can be used in different settings and with individuals who are in any position within an organisation.

This chapter describes what coaching is but also what it isn't. It then moves on to look at some of the skills you as an individual will find useful if you wish to develop a coaching mindset, have successful coaching conversations and enhance a coaching approach within your workplace. There are different types of coaching, which are described, with vignettes and examples to illustrate how these have been used in practice. These will demonstrate how powerful and transformational a coaching conversation can be. Following this, this chapter turns to the National Health Service (NHS), exploring the history of coaching in this environment. It asks, what, if any, embedding, has taken place, what form does it take and asks if it is really coaching. This chapter concludes with the impact that coaching can make,

D. Linay
ICF-Approved Professional Coach at Coaches in Mind (Self-employed),
London, England, United Kingdom
e-mail: Deniselinay@gmail.com

H. Rogers (✉)
ICF Approved Professional Coach at Coaches in Mind (self-employed), Ballina, Co Mayo, Eire
e-mail: Helen@helenrogerscoaching.com

© The Author(s), under exclusive license to Springer Nature Switzerland AG 2025
M. O'Brien, E. Kitson-Reynolds (eds.), *Respectful Relationships in the Maternity Service*, https://doi.org/10.1007/978-3-032-04281-1_5

the ripple effect that can be so powerful in the process of creating strong supportive cultures. It describes what to look for in a coach and how everyone can recognise a coaching opportunity and utilise those skills that will enable empowering conversations. Coaching is the 'golden thread of change' that can support individuals and teams to be the best that they can be. Where organisations embrace coaching, it can become a powerful tool to enable positive cultures to grow and develop and support healthy organisations to be even better.

## 5.2 So, What Is Coaching?

People are often familiar with the term coach, but usually in relation to sports coaching. When it comes to coaching individuals around career or personal goals, it isn't unusual to find that a more detailed explanation is needed because many people are unfamiliar with the term in this context; if it's the first time that they have met a coach, this is perfectly understandable. In any coaching relationship, the coachee may not be quite sure about what to expect and what benefits they will get out of the process. It is therefore important that they are given as much clear information as possible so that they can make informed choices as to what they want to achieve from coaching. Let's start by focusing on a simple explanation of coaching as a recognised process that has its roots in the world of sport but, which, over years, has evolved to be something less aligned to mentoring and which enables an individual to explore their values, beliefs and what might be stopping them from achieving their potential.

We believe, this is a clear explanation. Coaching is a process which can aid someone's development and assist them to be the best that they can be either in their personal or professional lives or both. Coaching can be about gaining confidence, progressing in their careers, or looking after their health and well-being; it is a process that can be adapted to many aspects of our lives. Even if someone decides to be coached to be the best they can be in a work context, they will discover that it also enables them to think about other aspects of their lives and vice versa. Good coaching takes a holistic approach, looking beyond a single aspect to explore other impacts. For example, someone who wants to be more organised and focused whilst at work will find that they bring those changes into their home life. This in turn can bring a better sense of balance in all parts of their lives so that they can be the best that they can be whatever life role they are in. Coachees are often surprised by this transferrable impact and by the positive results that they see at the end of a coaching relationship.

Unlike therapy or counselling, coaching is a forward-focused process. Of course, there will be times when previous experiences are referenced, but those experiences are not there to be interrogated. They help to make us who we are; coaching is not about dwelling on past experiences. The role of the coach is to assist the coachee in looking to the future, in setting goals and, by being useful, in getting them to the point where they are achievable. There will be questions and some challenges, but these are based on the belief that the coach trusts the coachee to find their own solutions, with the coachee trusting the coach to support them while they do so. The coach does not tell the coachee what they should and shouldn't do, as perhaps a mentor would, but rather by creating a safe supportive environment where the coach listens, and the coachee can think about what they want to achieve. This is a key aspect of coaching, and we are reminded by Nancy Kline, who in her book *Time to Think* describes how powerful, incisive listening can give people time and space to think; by doing this, thinking has the potential to be transformational (Kline 2002).

When discussing the coaching process, one of the first things that a coach will do is to assure the coachee that all their sessions are confidential. This is imperative if that safe supportive space is to be created and maintained. Of course, if coaching is commissioned, the manager, or another sponsor, they will want to see that goals have been met. It is important to set ground rules and boundaries with them and the coachee around this and any other disclosure issues before coaching commences.

There are many definitions of coaching, all are useful, but there is something sensible about keeping things simple so that prospective coachees are clear what they can expect and how a coach can be useful to them in achieving their goals. At present, coaching is unregulated. However, this does not mean that coaches should not be trained and accredited. It is possible to obtain internationally recognised qualifications through a recognised coaching body; it is important that anyone thinking of engaging a coach should ask whom they have trained with. It is also possible to ask if coaches are up to date with their continuing professional development and if they access coaching supervision. This is fundamental information that will help the coachee and coach to establish and build a trusting relationship, enabling them to work together in partnership. The two well-known coaching organisations are the International Coaching Federation (ICF) and the Association for Coaching (AC). Both recognised bodies provide accreditation for coach training and development as well as being membership organisations.

## 5.3    What Can You Expect from Coaching?

So, having said that coaching is a process, what can you expect from that process? As previously stated, coaching can be described as a future-focused conversation, which takes place in partnership. The coach facilitates the thinking of the coachee, or as Claire Pedrick, IFC, Master Certified Coach (MCC) describes them, the thinker, by creating a safe confidential space (Pedrick 2021). They will question and challenge in a supportive and appropriate manner, always with the aim of enabling the coachee to move forward to achieve whatever they want to.

Many staff come into the NHS because they want to help people, which is a common approach taken by healthcare staff. The Nursing and Midwifery Council (NMC) Standards for the Midwives (NMC 2019) encourage midwives to actively seek advice when unsure, to be helped to undertake tasks and problem solve. In practice, the expert practitioner shares experience, knowledge and skills with the novice, thus enabling them to be better practitioners. However, when it comes to coaching, a helpful coach may not serve a coachee well. Pedrick (2021) suggests that it is better to be useful rather than helpful, meaning it is better for the coach to let the coachee work out what they need to do for themselves rather than being told what to do. This provides ownership not only of the issue but also of the solution.

## 5.4    What Does the Process Look Like?

If the coach is a member of the ICF, they will be working to the core competencies of that organisation and the coachee can check these on the ICF website (International Coaching Federation 2025). First, the coach and coachee will agree if they want to work together; they will have a discovery conversation to make sure that they are a good fit for each other. This is important, as it is not possible to form a trusting relationship if this does not occur. It is totally acceptable for either one to say they believe the relationship will not work; this is not a poor reflection on either. Once they decide they can work together, they can move on to the 'how'. This is called contracting and is an important first stage, ensuring that both sides are clear about boundaries, confidentially and what is expected. There then follows a series of confidential conversations between coach and coachee. These conversations are based on mutual trust and respect where the former creates a safe, supportive but challenging space for the latter to explore, to grow and to develop thoughts and ideas. As previously stated, the coach does not tell the coachee what to do, they let them come to their own conclusions. It is a journey, and like all journeys, there may be diversions and bumps in the road. But it is what the individual learns on that journey that is often of more value than arriving at the destination. Coaching can be a transformational experience where the coachee learns who they really are and discovers their strengths, values and beliefs. They become more self-assured, more confident and have the courage to be the best that they can be. They often go on to be positive role models for other staff and colleagues.

Coaching is a relationship where collaboration and partnership are key; otherwise, it simply will not work. The coach comes to that relationship believing that the coachee wants to be there, that they want to achieve whatever goals they set and are prepared to do their best to achieve this. The coach is responsible for providing a supportive, confidential space. The coachee's responsibility is to fully engage and take responsibility for any agreed actions. It is a relationship where those who fully engage in the process reap the benefits, those who for whatever reason, do not, will not see the value of coaching. Basically, you get out of it what you put in. Coaching can be confused with counselling or therapy, whilst in recent years, there is more of a merging with therapy, which is not the same thing (Starr 2021). Coaching does not aim to treat any psychological problems. A coachee will always be told that it is their responsibility to disclose any professional treatment that they may have had or be receiving. This does not mean that coaching will be stopped, but it may be suspended if a professional intervention is more appropriate. There may also be times when it is appropriate for a coach to suggest referral to relevant services. Now that we have talked about what coaching is, we can move on to what skills are important for anyone who would like to develop a coaching mindset and culture.

## 5.5 Coaching Conversation Skills and Developing a Coaching Mindset

Attention is the rarest and purest form of generosity (Weil 1948). There is nothing mystical about developing a coaching mindset. It simply involves utilising the communication skills that make us human. Unfortunately, in our busy lives, these skills can become dulled. The good news is that practising them will inevitably improve both your professional and personal relationships, increase your influence and contribute to a psychologically safe workplace environment for yourself, your colleagues and service users. This section will focus on the skills needed for a coaching conversation. It is not intended to fully equip you to be a coach, nor will it cover all skills coaches receive training in. However, it will support you in developing a coaching mindset and to encourage those you work alongside to also do so. Numerous books have been written on coaching, a few of which have been cited in this chapter (Kline 2002; Whitmore 2009; Starr 2008, 2011, 2021; Pedrick 2021); while they often reference the same core skills, there are some differences in how these skills are described. For our purposes, the skills identified below will be covered:

1. Listening to understand
2. Questioning
3. Playback
4. Feedback
5. The use of silence
6. Empathy

At first glance, you might think that some of these aren't really skills. But stay with it.

### 5.5.1 Listening to Understand

Have you ever met up with a friend and left feeling deflated or exhausted, without quite knowing why? Or perhaps you had a nagging feeling that you dominated the conversation. In either case, it's possible that you weren't truly listening or being listened to. As Stephen Covey, author of *The 7 Habits of Highly Effective People*, famously said, 'Most people do not listen with the intent to understand; they listen with the intent to reply' (Covey 2004). Definitions of listening vary from 'To give attention with the ear to some sound or utterance' (Oxford English Dictionary [OED] 2024) to Burt's more considered view that it 'encompasses all the ways in which a listener becomes aware of what a speaker is experiencing and expressing in a given moment' (Burt 2019, p. 3).

Experiencing and expressing is not just about paying attention to the words being said. Covey (2004) noted that only 10% of our communication is represented by the words we use, the remaining 90% is expressed by our sounds and body language.

There are various levels of listening, ranging from superficial to deep, with different writers describing these levels in various ways. Figure 5.1 compares the approaches of two such writers.

If you ask someone, 'How are you?' and they respond with, 'I'm good', the way they say it gives you additional information. Is their tone upbeat or despondent? Does their body language match their words? If their 'I'm good' doesn't align with their tone or body language, how do you respond? Your response will likely depend on your relationship with the person. A casual acquaintance may only receive a quick nod, while a colleague, friend, or relative may prompt you to inquire further. As Whitmore aptly observes in *Coaching for Performance*, 'When the words say one thing, but the body seems to say something else, the body is more likely to indicate the true feelings' (Whitmore 2009, p. 50).

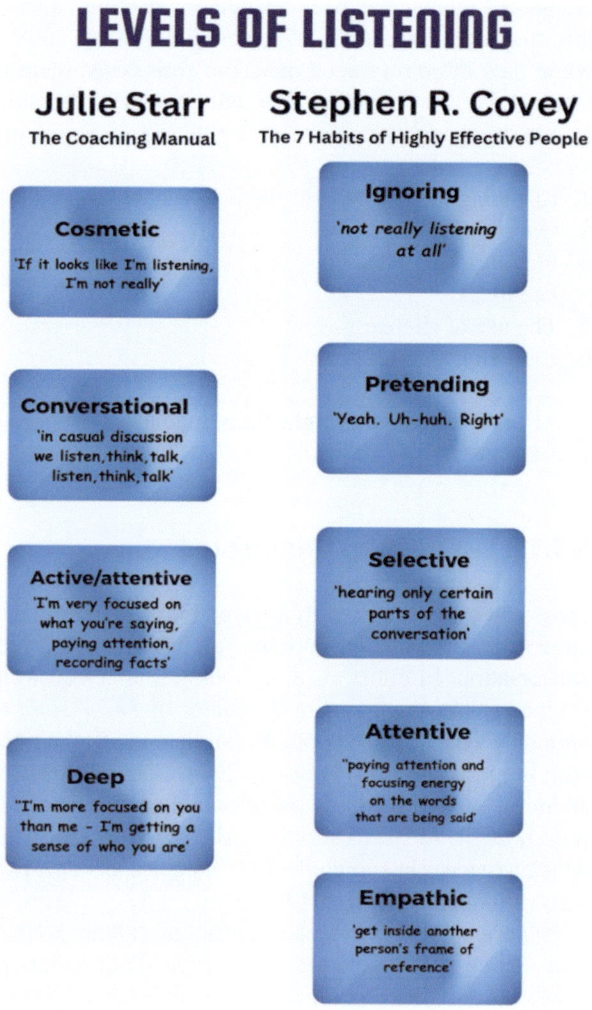

**Fig. 5.1** The levels of listening

What should be clear is that there is no right or wrong level of listening, it depends on the situation. Engaging with a stranger in a queue may only require a superficial or 'pretending' level of listening. However, speaking to a distressed colleague demands a much deeper level of attention, as failure to listen at this higher level could heighten their distress. While not being listened to can be mildly irritating when you're casually complaining about the length of a queue, it can have a far greater impact when you need to connect, whether to discuss a troubling event or share good news. Many coaches, when they begin their training, become more aware of situations where they aren't being truly listened to. This heightened awareness can affect their personal relationships. Do they still want to meet up with someone who only talks at them? Perhaps not. This realisation can stir challenging emotions, but becoming more conscious of when you're not being listened to will, in turn, help you improve your own listening skills (Fig. 5.2).

In a coaching conversation, listening to the speaker requires your full attention. Just as you listen not only by hearing the words but by noticing how they are said and observing body language, the speaker will notice the same about you. Are you holding eye contact? Is your body *open* i.e. your arms are not crossed? Are you subtly mirroring the tone of voice and body language of the speaker? Mirroring body language will create a stronger sense of connection. For example, if the speaker leans forward leaning forward too will strengthen the connection, but leaning back could break it. Any movement needs to be subtle and natural; if it is obvious, it may be perceived as intimidation.

## 5.5.2 Questioning

If you're truly listening to understand, rather than just to respond, you'll naturally have questions. Asking a question sends a clear signal that you're listening and interested in knowing more. Of course, in a casual conversation, you might ask a question simply to be polite. For example, if someone in the queue mentions they're going on holiday, you may ask where they're going. Their response might deepen the conversation, or it might not.

When talking with a friend, you'll likely ask questions out of genuine interest. If they mention a holiday destination you're also interested in, you may ask about how they booked it or what the cost was. Alternatively, they might tell you they're considering applying for a job, and you might inquire about where they saw the listing because it piques your own interest. Sometimes, we ask questions just to be nosy, and these conversations are easily recognisable. However, in a coaching conversation, the role of the coach is to '*serve the speaker*' (Burt 2009, p. 36). When a conversation shifts from mutual interest to a focus on the speaker, you are entering into a coaching conversation. In a coaching session, a coach will first ask questions to understand the issue the coachee wants to discuss. The coach doesn't need to become an expert on the issue, but should understand enough to move the conversation forward. For example, if the coachee mentions they're thinking of applying for

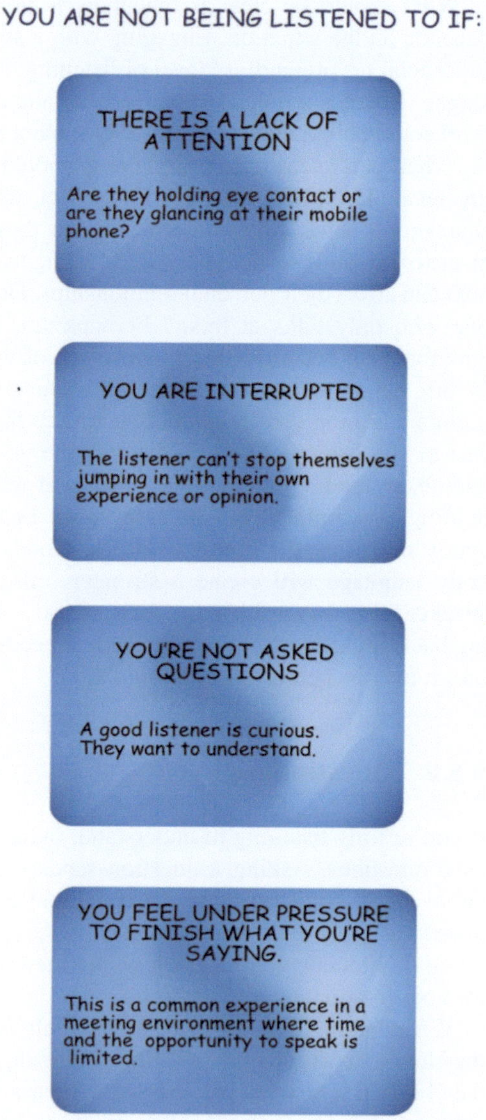

**Fig. 5.2** Signs you are not being listened to (courtesy of Denise Linay)



a job, the coach won't ask where the job was advertised, as that is likely to be irrelevant.

One of the idiosyncrasies of offering coaching is that potential coachees often seek a coach with expertise in their specific field. However, as Whitmore notes, this can lead to what he calls the *'pitfalls of knowledge'* where experts find it difficult 'to withhold their expertise sufficiently to coach well' (Whitmore 2009, p. 42). He recounts a situation where, due to the overbooking of Inner Tennis courses, he brought in two Inner Ski coaches, dressed them in tennis attire and handed them tennis rackets. Surprisingly, though not to Whitmore 'the coaching job they performed was largely indistinguishable from that of their tennis-playing colleagues'. In fact, on a few occasions, they even did a better job. Upon reflection, it became clear that while the tennis coaches focused on correcting technical faults, the ski coaches paid attention to how efficiently the participants used their bodies. This allowed them to address the root cause of the problem, whereas the tennis coaches were only addressing the symptoms. As a result, the tennis coaches needed extra training to help them detach from their technical expertise.

Once the coach understands the issue, further questions focus on deepening the coachee's understanding of their situation. Effective questions, often referred to by commentators, are open-ended, requiring the coachee to think more deeply. For example, instead of asking 'Do you feel upset when your manager speaks to you that way?', which seeks a yes/no response and also suggests how the coachee should feel, the coach might ask, 'How do you feel when your manager speaks to you in that way?', which invites the coachee to reflect more deeply on their emotions.

> **Box 5.1 Exercise: Do I Really Listen?**
>
> Can you think of a situation where it was obvious that your manager and/or colleague was not listening to you?
>
> How does this make you feel?
>
> Do you believe that you listen effectively to colleagues and/or staff? What could you do differently to improve your listening skills?

> **Box 5.2 Vignette—Moving from Understanding the Situation to Asking the Effective Question**
>
> Jane is upset. She has just had a meeting with her manager to discuss a leadership post she has applied for; her manager's reaction to this has made her feel that she should withdraw her application.
>
> You ask her a couple of questions to understand the background to the conversation.
>
> Once you have a sufficient understanding of the situation, you could ask 'If you were the manager how would you have handled the meeting?' This has the potential to move Jane away from the negative impact of the meeting to consider and acknowledge that she has the leadership qualities that make her eligible to apply for the post.

It's important to ask one question at a time. In everyday conversation, we often ask multiple questions at once or rephrase the same question in different ways if we feel it wasn't clear the first time. However, in coaching, it's important to be comfortable with silence and take time to think before asking the next question. There is some debate about using 'why' questions in coaching. While 'why' can sometimes come across as demanding justification, in a softer tone, it can open the conversation. Ultimately, it depends on how it's asked.

### 5.5.3  Playback and Feedback

> **Box 5.3 Vignette—Giving Effective Playback**
>
> In everyday conversations, it's not uncommon for listeners to play back or summarise what they've heard, especially if they've momentarily lost focus. Sometimes, playback is followed by an opinion, which may or may not be helpful. For example:
>
> John has been job hunting for months and finally has an interview, but he's anxious. In a conversation with his friend, he jumps into a lengthy account all the reasons why he should turn the interview down. His friend, familiar with John's self-doubt, might respond with 'So you've got an interview, but you're thinking of turning it down because you don't feel ready? Don't be so stupid'.
>
> His friend may have effectively summarised the lengthy account John has given, and this may be enough for John, when hearing the playback, to think 'I'm being stupid'. But his friend referring to him as being stupid may come across as dismissive and do little to challenge John's self-limiting beliefs.

In coaching, the response would be different. Firstly, the coach would give John the space to consider the summary of his situation. If he agrees it is an accurate account, the coach may ask 'Can you tell me more about why you don't feel ready?' or 'What does "ready" feel like to you?' This encourages John to reflect more deeply and potentially challenge his own assumptions. Alternately, John may dispute the coach's summary, which again can lead to a wider and/or deeper conversation. Effective playback also demonstrates active listening. By using the coachee's keywords and phrases, you show that you've truly understood them. If you substitute their words with different ones, they may feel misunderstood, even if the meaning is the same to you.

Feedback is aimed at developing self-awareness. In listening to the speaker, the coach may have observed the speaker being very judgemental of themselves or others, the continued use of a phrase such as 'am I making myself clear' or a change in their tone of voice when speaking about something or someone. Providing feedback is a judgement call and has to be sensitively handled. A coach will often ask permission of the speaker before they give the feedback.

> **Box 5.4 Vignette—Giving Effective Feedback**
>
> Nishma is a newly qualified coach. She is still in a full-time job in teaching, but is considering reducing her hours to develop a coaching practice. The issue she wanted to be coached on was her coaching niche. She had identified a number of options, the easiest and, possibly, the most lucrative was to coach headteachers. But when she spoke about this niche, she sounded flat, whereas when she spoke about her other options, she sounded more upbeat, even excited. The coach tells Nishma that she noticed changes in her energy when she speaks about prospective niches and asks her if she is happy to hear what has been observed. Nishma agrees.
>
> On hearing the coach's feedback, there was silence. Nishma was thinking. Eventually, she responded, admitting that coaching headteachers did not excite her, although she had not acknowledged this until the coach made the observation. However, it was a group that was more likely to pay for her services and one that she was already in contact with. This led to a more productive conversation about taking her coaching business forward.

## 5.5.4 The Use of Silence

Silence can feel uncomfortable in a conversation and is often seen as a lack of communication or even a breakdown in the relationship (Burt 2019, p.57). We often feel compelled to fill silences, a tactic police use effectively during interrogations to prompt confessions. Silence can be incredibly powerful. When we're alone with our thoughts, it often leads to insights and new ideas. The same applies in conversations. A pause doesn't mean someone has stopped thinking; it often signals they are processing what was said. As a coach, one of the most undervalued skills is the ability to embrace silence. Overcoming the discomfort of silence gives the coachee time to reflect and think more deeply. The coach listens to the quiet, not knowing what the coachee is thinking, but trusting that they are, until they are ready to speak again.

## 5.5.5 Empathy

> Empathy is our ability to identify what someone else is thinking or feeling, and to respond to their thoughts and feelings with an appropriate emotion. (Baron-Cohen 2012, p. 12)

This definition suggests that there are two stages in empathy: recognition and response. Listening and understanding the experience of another person constitutes the recognition stage; how you respond is where you build trust. It's important here to distinguish between empathy, sympathy and compassion. A number of writers stress the importance of not showing sympathy when coaching Starr states that sympathy involves sharing another person's feelings, while empathy is about understanding those feelings without necessarily taking them on (Starr 2011). Brene

Brown goes further, describing sympathy as 'the near enemy of empathy' (Brown 2021, p. 124), noting that it has the potential to trigger shame.

In coaching, empathy allows the coach to remain objective and impartial while still connecting deeply with the coachee's experience. Compassion, on the other hand, is empathy in action, understanding someone's pain and taking steps to alleviate it. However, a coach's role is not to rescue the coachee, but to support them in finding their own solutions. An example of where your empathy can tip over to rescue is when someone becomes tearful during a coaching conversation. You may feel compelled to apologise for making them cry and steer the conversation away from the issue that has upset them. But being able to cry is a human characteristic. No other animal can cry. It has the potential to lessen the body of physical and mental pain and increases our ability to think. So not only do we need to get comfortable with silence if we are going to coach well but we also need to become comfortable with tears.

It is important to recognise that just like the other skills of coaching, empathy needs to be practised. For some people, it happens easily, but for others, it can be more challenging. Baron-Cohen claims that we *all lie somewhere on an empathy spectrum'* (Baron-Cohen 2012, p. 11). And it is a skill that can be eroded if we are continually having to deal with a stressful work environment. The introduction to this chapter referred to the importance of contracting in coaching. This is the process of ensuring that the coach and the coachee are 'a good fit'. There are a number of reasons why it may not be a good fit and sometimes the reason is difficult to articulate. It just doesn't feel right. But it may be that the views on a particular issue or issues are diametrically opposed. Climate change is a commonly cited issue, which can invoke strong views. If a coach feels that they would find it difficult to empathise with the coachee, they would have to consider not entering into the contract. In a coaching conversation, you may experience triggers that test how empathetic you feel towards the person you are speaking to, but it may be enough to just acknowledge the emotion you are feeling whilst keeping your attention.

Now is probably a good time to recognise that coaching conversations can be tiring. It would be impossible to go from one coaching conversation to another, maintaining the same level of attention that is required. Whilst developing a coaching mindset and being able to have coaching conversations is going to benefit you, your colleagues and service users, you need a mix of other interactions and, occasionally, some quiet time to yourself to re-energise.

Finally, this section opened with a Simone Weil quote that 'attention is the rarest and purest form of generosity' (Weil 1948). The skills described in this section and the following five top tips will support you to give others the attention they need to flourish (Fig. 5.3).

**Fig. 5.3** Five top tips for achieving full attention

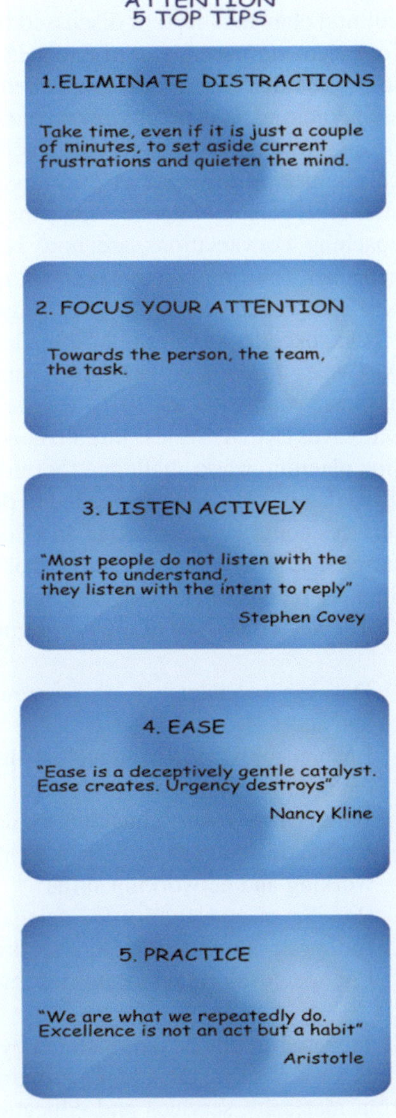


## 5.6    Coaching for Leadership

The legendary American football coach Vince Lombardi once said, 'Leaders aren't born, they are made. And they are made just like anything else, through hard work'.

People learn and develop over time and by experience. They may have traits that will help them to be great leaders, but it is often the situations that they find themselves in that make them who they are. Coaching has previously been identified as a 'golden thread of change' (see Sect. 1.5). Its impotany contribution to achieving cultural change is further discussed in the final chapter (see Chap. 8). It may therefore seem surprising that in the NHS and maternity services there is little evidence to suggest that coaching is embedded or offered routinely to staff to develop leadership potential. If coaching is offered, it appears to be to those who are, or aspire to be, in senior management positions. This is a missed opportunity. The time to offer coaching is at the start of an individual's career so that they can build on their strengths, gain confidence and be the leaders they want to be. There is evidence that coaching conversations are now being integrated into midwifery training programmes, for example, this is something that Welsh universities offer as part of their NMC-approved pre-registration midwifery education programmes (NMC 2023).

One excellent example of a leadership programme, which does just this, is the All-Wales Midwifery Leadership and Development Programme (MLDP), which has been running since 2016. This is a joint Welsh Government and Royal College Midwives (RCM) Wales' initiative, which was triggered by recognising that succession planning was a challenge for midwifery leadership. Alongside this, it was identified that investment was needed to develop midwives at all levels so that maternity services could be delivered at an effective high-quality level. The result has been a simple and low-cost programme that has now been expanded to include Maternity Support Workers (MSWs).

The key objectives of the programme are to:

- Develop a leadership programme that was people focused, easy to deliver and access
- Enable midwives to develop their leadership skills in a safe, supportive environment
- Provide one-to-one coaching for delegates
- Enable delegates to undertake a project to develop and experience collaborative working and networking skills
- Provide an opportunity for delegates to join future steering groups in order to further develop their leadership skills
- Provide coaching opportunities for midwives

The programme is administered by a steering group that is made up of the RCM Director for Wales, the Chief Midwife from Welsh Government and representatives from maternity services and education, all of whom have been previous participants. This gives them the opportunity to further develop their leadership skills. The programme is supported by Heads of Midwifery (HOMs), Directors of Midwifery (DOMs) and Directors of Nursing (DONs), as well as the RCM, Welsh Government Ministers and the Chief Nursing Officer (CNO) for Wales. The steering group plans the annual programme and ensures that the objectives are met. It runs over a six-month period and delegates are invited to apply to their HOM/DOM so that they may be considered for a place. They then attend four study days and a final showcase day. At the outset, they are asked to present an idea to the delegate group and projects are picked following a presentation and voting process. Delegates from across the country work together to deliver the project that they then present at the showcase day via the medium of a poster. The key element that makes this programme stand out is that each delegate is paired with a coach for the duration. The emphasis is not on the project, but rather on what they have learned about themselves over the 6 months. They are invited to think about their strengths and skills and what kind of leaders they are. The coaches are chosen from the maternity services, and support is given to them to build on coaching techniques. Whilst not all the coaches are qualified, the aim is to grow a culture where coaching language and techniques are utilised and become the norm. Each delegate gives a 10-min presentation at the showcase day where they share their leadership journey and what they have learned along the way.

Historically, the programme cohort has consisted of delegates from the midwifery workforce; however, last-year MSWs were included. The programme has been seen to be successful and feedback from delegates and coaches has been very positive. Many of the delegates have gone on to gain more senior leadership roles. The programme is also now a case study for the World Health Organisation (WHO) European roadmap (WHO 2021).

## 5.7    Coaching for Career Development

Coaching can be a powerful tool in assisting an individual to plan and progress in their career. The process can give an individual a framework within which they can identify their strengths and what they might need to build on to think about what their next career move might be. Working with a coach can also give them the space that they need to reflect on their own values, on who they are and what drives them. This can be invaluable when they are considering where to go next. A coach will also work with that individual so that they build confidence in their ability to apply, attend interview and get the job that they want.

**Box 5.5 Vignette—Coaching for Career Development**
Jo was at a crossroads in her career. She had applied for several posts, which would give her the promotion that she craved, but had been consistently unsuccessful. A colleague suggested that she might benefit from coaching. At the discovery session, Jo acknowledged that she was feeling frustrated and had lost confidence in herself. She stated that she did not know where to go next.

Prior to the first session, the coach asked Jo to do some exercises. These were a life map and a strengths exercise. The life map gave Jo a vehicle to look back on her life and identify the highs and lows, whilst the strengths one asked her to record what she was good at. When she arrived at the first session, she talked about how useful both exercises had been. She had forgotten

(continued)

**Box 5.5** (continued)

that she had achieved a great deal in her life and career and how good that felt. She also remarked that drafting her life map had reminded her of how she had reacted to and learnt from some to the less positive experiences. She found that listing her strengths was quite challenging, and it was easier for her to say what she was not good at.

This session proved to be a turning point for Jo. She embraced coaching with a positive mindset and subsequent conversations also enabled her to reflect on her values, on what made her who she was and where she wanted to go in her career. As a result, she was able to identify a job that she really wanted to do and that fitted her leadership style. With her coach's support she applied, was interviewed and appointed to her dream job.

## 5.8  Coaching for Wellness

*'You can't pour from an empty cup',* says the old proverb. And it is true that you need to take care of yourself first.

When someone accesses a coach, it is often for one specific issue, whether it be around leadership, confidence building or career development. It would be a mistake, however, to think that the issue they come with can be seen in isolation from everything else. The coachee may want to think about how they can be their best in a new job, for instance. However, they will always bring something of themselves into the conversation. They are not just Mary the manager of a busy department. They may also be a mother, daughter, sister, wife, partner, friend or colleague. The manager part of them might be the initial focus, but if they put all their energy into succeeding as that, they may find there is nothing left to give to the other components in their lives.

It is often much easier to think through an issue such as being successful at interview and to set goals to achieve this. When it comes to wellness, however, this is often much harder. This is evident in the setting of New Year resolutions, whether they are about losing weight, getting fitter or quitting smoking. The intention is sound, and many make it to the starting line, which is why, by the end of January, we often see adverts offering exercise bikes which are as good as new. In his book, *Atomic Habits*, James Clear states that it can 'take 66 days before a new behaviour becomes automatic' (Clear 2018). He quotes a study by Phillipa Lally, a health psychology researcher at University College London and published in the European Journal of Social Psychology (Lally et al. 2010). Lally's study found that it took between 18 and 254 days for people to form a new habit. This suggests that habits take time to form, to be embedded, and this is where coaching has a huge role to play. Coaching can help individuals to work out priorities, make space for themselves and find a sense of balance so that they can make sure that there is something in the cup for everyone, but most importantly, that there is something there for themselves.

**Box 5.6 Vignette—Finding Balance**

Mary had decided that she would benefit from accessing coaching. She had a busy full-time job that she loved. It was also a very important aspect of her life, and she wanted to be the best manager that she could possibly be. The discovery session went well, and Mary and her coach agreed that they would work together. Mary came to the first session, saying that she would like to think about her time management. She wanted more control over her diary and wanted to be more productive at work. As time went on, Mary started to recognise that she did very little outside of work, and, worst of all, she did nothing for herself. She was feeling stressed, tired and anxious about letting people down when she said no to invitations. And she was conscious that she had put on weight and could not remember when she last took some serious exercise.

In the third session, Mary suddenly sat back and declared that she wanted to change her goal. She felt that the balance between work and family was not right and that she would like it to be better. She wanted to be fit and healthy. She wanted to enjoy her work but not to the extent that it was all consuming. In essence, she had taken a holistic view of her life, and she did not like what she saw. So, the first thing that the coach did was to ask Mary what she would like to see that was different. She was encouraged to look at herself 2 years hence and describe what she would see if things were different. Mary saw someone who was fit and healthy, who loved her job but who also had a meaningful social and family life. She saw someone who had balance. As a result, Mary started to think about how this could be achieved. She had always thought that she should put everyone else's needs before her own and felt guilty if she put herself first.

Through coaching, she learned that it was ok to put herself first sometimes; indeed, if she did not, she would not be able to look after others. With the support of her coach, she set small achievable goals around her health and well-being. These included putting time aside to go for a walk, to go cycling with her husband and to leave work on time. Like all good habits, Mary had good and less good days, but she learned that the more she worked on these, the easier and more embedded they became. She did one very simple thing at the end of each day; she thought about one positive thing that had happened, either at work or elsewhere. This started as an internal exercise but soon she found that she was telling her family around the dinner table, and they were giving her their examples as well. Mary reached the end of her coaching journey and told her coach that for the first time in years she was happier and healthier, that she had found balance.

## 5.9    Coaching to Deal with a Workplace Issue

A common reason for someone to consider coaching is when they are experiencing problems at work. A coach can provide a safe, supportive space to explore the issue, challenge any self-limiting beliefs that may be keeping them 'stuck' and work with them to find a solution.

> **Box 5.7 Vignette—Dealing with a Workplace Issue**
>
> Louisa was struggling. She was in a senior post, leading a team but was being undermined and micromanaged by her direct line manager. This situation had been going on for a while, which was having a detrimental impact on Louisa's confidence.
>
> During the first coaching session, Louisa told the coach that she felt stuck. She couldn't deal with the way her manager treated her, but did not have the confidence to look for another job.
>
> This isn't unusual. People often put up with situations that gradually erode their self-worth. By the time they decide to do something about it, there is a fair amount of rebuilding to do.
>
> The coach explored with Louisa how she reacted to her manager's actions. Her manager often sent her long emails that listed actions she wanted her to take. They didn't need a response, but Louisa felt compelled to reply particularly if the email was critical of her.
>
> What would happen if Louisa didn't reply? After some thought, Louisa said, 'nothing'. She agreed that this was an action she could sign up to.
>
> On her return, Louisa had only replied to those emails that required a response. She had resisted replying to the others. She felt that she was taking control, she was not thinking about the contents of the emails as much and, interestingly, she wasn't being sent as many.
>
> Whilst it is often true that you cannot change the behaviour of others as you can only change how you respond, sometimes, that response can bring about a change.
>
> Louisa started feeling more confident in herself as a leader. A few months later, she successfully applied for a more senior position in another organisation.

## 5.10    Team Coaching

In his book, *The Definitive Guide to Team Coaching*, David Clutterbuck quotes Katzenbach and Smith (1999), who define a team as:

> A small number of people with complementary skills, who are committed to a common purpose, performance goals and approach, for which they hold themselves mutually accountable' calling it 'one of the most commonly quoted definitions to describe what a team is. (Clutterbuck 2007)

Maternity services are familiar with the team concept whether that is in the hospital or community services. Staff will have complementary skills, be they doctors, managers, midwives or support staff. Their goals and approaches will be the same in relation to caring for women and families and the team will be mutually accountable in ensuring safe effective services. Just as there is little evidence that coaching has been embedded in the NHS, there is also very little to suggest that team coaching is being used.

Team coaching can be an important component of teambuilding. It can enable a new or existing team to gel and perform to their best ability. As in any coaching relationship, it is important to establish the purpose before any coaching takes place. This may happen with the team manager or sponsor, but everyone should recognise that this is just an exploratory general discussion. The team members will want and be able to have input and ownership of the process at as early a stage as possible. If this does not happen, there is a danger that it could feel like a 'done to' process that is unlikely to get positive results. This may also be an indication of what the organisational culture is like. Hierarchical cultures that take a top-down approach may be less likely to involve those staff who are seen to be at a lower level. This is not likely to generate trust and engagement amongst staff. Clear ground rules and confidentiality are key in any coaching relationship, but are especially important when it involves a team. The coach in this scenario will work with the team, enabling them to build a strong purposeful unit; they will also help them to grow as individuals. Successful teams will have a high level of trust and respect for each other. They will support each other and will have each other's best interests at heart. This, in turn, can enable the team to provide safe, effective care.

## 5.11 Coaching Through Action Learning Sets

Another way for a coach to work with a small number of people is by facilitating an Action Learning Set (ALS). In their book, *Action Learning: A Practitioner's Guide*, Ian McGill and Liz Beaty describe Action Learning as 'a process of learning and reflection that happens with the support of a group or 'Set' of colleagues working with real problems with the intention of getting things done' (McGill and Beaty 1992). There is very little written about ALS in relation to midwifery. However, it was used as a learning tool in the preparation of Supervisors of Midwives until that model was changed in 2017.

A facilitator enables the presenter to set the scene and then the set coaches the presenter by asking questions and challenging assumptions. At the end of the session, the presenter will aim to have an action plan to take forward. The set takes responsibility to keep the presenter safe and they can learn by reflection and thinking about new approaches. No one tells the presenter what to do. Instead, they are encouraged through questioning to find their own solutions. The set members bring real issues to explore and take it in turns to present what they want to think about. ALS works well because it is run by the set for the set. Everyone has time to present and question in any given session and they can run over several weeks or months. A coach can act as facilitator to the set and will ensure that the presenter gets what they need from their session. An ALS approach can help organisations to change culture, as it relies on them to be less hierarchical and encourages them to have a more open approach to dealing with mistakes. Those organisations may take longer to embrace ALS, and this is where a coach can make a huge difference. They will encourage a coaching approach and mindset amongst the set, which can then grow in confidence. The coach can encourage the members to trust and respect each other and enable them to grow and develop to the point where they manage themselves and no longer need a coach.

## 5.12    Coaching in Healthcare

Coaching is not new in healthcare, though its use varies significantly across regions and organisations. Even within a single organisation, coaching practices may differ widely. In addition, some interventions may utilise coaching skills without them being explicitly referred to as such; alternatively, the term 'coaching' may be mistakenly applied to other interventions, most notably, mentoring. Despite the widespread acknowledgement of the benefits of coaching, embraced by organisations like Google™, Coca-Cola™ and Microsoft™, some still view it as a non-essential service to be discarded when budgets are tight or to be reserved for senior leaders such as Chief Executive Officers. Whilst there is increasing evidence that the NHS is investing in coaching (NHS Leadership Academy 2025a, b; Sinclair et al. 2008; Iordanou et al. 2017) as a key strategy for performance improvement, there isn't yet the evidence that would suggest that it is receiving the same investment as it does in other organisations.

Access to coaching is also likely to be different across the four UK countries. For example, the NHS Leadership Academy claims on its Coaching and Mentoring Hub that 'coaching and mentoring is an inclusive offering available to all professions within the NHS and Social Care irrespective of pay grade, clinical and non-clinical roles' (NHS Leadership Academy 2025a, b). This offer is in England only; although it claims to work collaboratively across the four nations of the UK, the comparable organisations in Wales, Scotland and Northern Ireland don't have the same explicit offer. There is also no data available on the uptake of the offer made by the NHS Leadership Academy, nor what is meant by the term 'professions'. What we do know is that the use of coaching in maternity was being referred to over 20 years ago. *The Bullying Culture*, a book that explored the causes of bullying, its effect and how it could be reduced in midwifery, recognised that 'coaching is an unexplored source for potential development' (Hadikin and O'Driscoll 2000, p. 152), which could be used to address bullying behaviour. The authors claim that it can:

> make a real difference in developing these individuals so that they can move forward and be contributing members of the team once more. (Hadikin and O'Driscoll 2000, p. 157)

However, whilst any intervention that helps to resolve issues without resorting to a formal process is to be applauded, this association with problem behaviour can give coaching a negative reputation, as something imposed as punishment rather than as a developmental tool.

Most studies on coaching in the NHS focus on its use in supporting senior leaders, its introduction in individual organisations, across development programmes and the teaching of students. Unfortunately, there is a lack of evidence that captures the incidence of coaching across the NHS as a whole and the similarities and differences between different countries, regions, organisations and workplaces. One of the challenges of undertaking such a review is that coaching is sometimes confused with mentoring and whilst they should complement each other, they are not the same. For example, a study carried out in 2013, *Practical coaching by mentors: Student Midwives' perceptions*, (Finnerty and Collington 2013) made no reference to the use of coaching skills, focusing exclusively on how mentors used techniques to help students access their craft knowledge. This was undoubtedly due to the researchers using a definition of coaching that is applied in sport coaching (see Sect. 5.2). Hopefully, our understanding of what is meant by coaching has moved on since that study with organisations like the NHS Leadership Academy (2025a, b) making very clear distinctions as to what is meant by coaching and mentoring:

> Coaching involves using questioning and inquiry to help individuals unlock their potential and achieve personal and professional success. Mentoring focuses on developing individuals by sharing knowledge, skills, and experience. (NHS Leadership Academy 2025a, b)

A more recent study (Thomas 2022) in the British Journal of Midwifery explored the use of both coaching and mentoring skills in complementing the Professional Midwifery Advocate (PMA) role, particularly around restorative clinical supervision. The study identified the shared features and distinctions between coaching and mentoring, highlighting the need for PMA's 'to have an increased awareness with regard to their coachee's body language' a clear nod to the use of coaching skills. Undoubtedly, the skills of coaching and mentoring complement each other. A mentor who employs coaching skills like active listening, open questioning and effective feedback will cultivate a trusting relationship that will support midwives and student midwives to find their own solutions, increase their resilience and improve their critical thinking. Studies such as this may suggest that coaching is becoming a universal approach to staff development and professional growth, but this isn't reflected on the public facing websites of regulatory and professional organisations operating in the NHS. For example, a review of NMC documents makes it difficult to know if the NMC supports coaching, with any references to it almost exclusively confined to the Register of Interests.

In addition to coaching being used to develop NHS staff, there is an increased use of health coaching to support patients with, or at risk of, one or more long-term condition(s), reflecting a broader shift from a traditional *doing to* model of care to a more collaborative *doing with* approach (Iordanou et al. 2017). However, whilst there is a growing body of evidence of health coaching being used in maternity services, this is predominantly from countries outside of the UK, for example, in Australia, all pregnant women have access to coaching sessions through the 'Get Healthy in Pregnancy' programme (Get Healthy Service New South Wales 2025).

There are a number of NHS policies/initiatives where the skills of coaching are deployed to the benefit of patients, although they are not always labelled and recognised as such. An example of this is the NHS initiative, Making Every Contact Count (MECC) (Public Health England 2016). This is an NHS policy introduced in 2008 designed to encourage behaviour change through everyday interactions between healthcare professionals and patients. While NHS documents on MECC don't specify the skills required to have these positive interactions, a number of publications do refer to the use of coaching skills. For instance, a factsheet discussing the use of healthy conversation skills (Infant and Toddler Forum 2019) mentions using '*open discovery questions*' and '*spending more time listening than providing information*'. Lawrence et al. (2016 p. 3) undertook an evaluation of MECC in 2016, describing the use of *exploratory conversations* in which practitioners attempt to understand patients' perspectives and help them plan their own solutions, with activities closely aligned with coaching principles, even though not explicitly labelled as such. Although MECC remains NHS policy (NHS Standard Contract 2023–24), there is evidence that many NHS employees are unaware of it. A 2018 national survey of 1387 NHS health professionals (Keyworth et al. 2018) found that only 31.4% had heard of MECC, although 55.9% recognised a need to provide opportunistic behaviour change interventions. Yet, in half of the cases where a need was perceived, no intervention was delivered, highlighting a gap between awareness and action. Other interventions in the maternity setting that utilise coaching skills are motivational interviewing and social prescribing. Both these approaches seek to support patients in managing their own health conditions particularly where there is an ambivalence or resistance to behaviour change.

In summary, while coaching is increasingly recognised in healthcare, its application varies and misconceptions persist. More research is needed to explore its full potential, especially for frontline staff, and to distinguish it more clearly from related practices like mentoring whilst at the same time acknowledge the importance of coaching skills inherent in the delivery of health policy and initiatives.

## 5.13    The Ripple Effect of Coaching

> Coaching is not a technique to be learnt, but a way of being, a way of managing, a way of treating people, a way of thinking, a way of being. (Whitmore 2009)

Coaching is increasingly recognised as integral to an organisation's strategy in leadership development and performance improvement as well as in improving employee engagement and retention. However, access to coaching is unlikely in the immediate future to be available to all healthcare workers. This may be due to a range of factors: the value their manager puts on coaching, the culture of the organisation, their pay grade or just the sheer size of the NHS workforce. The NHS in the UK employs 1.7 million people. It is the fifth biggest employer in the world. If every employee was offered an hour of coaching per year that equates to just over 45,332 weeks. So, if access to formal coaching is just not possible in an organisation the size of the NHS where resources are limited, a greater focus needs to be made on capitalising on the impact it has had on those who have had formal coaching. The Association for Coaching in its Vision and Purpose refers to the ripple effect:

> Our Vision is to professionalise and advance coaching, promoting a coach approach to leadership so coaching 'ripples' as a key enabler for performance, responsibility and fulfillment. (Association for Coaching n.d.-a, b)

But what is meant by the ripple effect? Is it, for example, the benefits that others experience as a consequence of their managers becoming better leaders or is it that the coachee starts to mirror their coaching experience in their conversations with others? Or is it a combination of both? First, it needs to be established whether a ripple effect does exist. It may seem evident that when a leader receives coaching, the benefits extend beyond the individual, impacting those they lead. This was confirmed in a recent study which found that 91% of direct reports observed a positive impact from their leader's coaching (Weingarten 2023, p. 2). However, an earlier study reported a *decline in the perceived quality of interactions* between others and those who had been coached (O'Connor and Cavanagh 2013, p. 1). In Coaching that Counts, Anderson and Anderson (2005) refer to the cascading effect of each successful coaching engagement '*creating positive change beyond the person receiving the coaching*' (p. 19). This suggests that it is the quality of the coaching that determines the impact it has on others.

Unfortunately, there is limited research on the ripple effect of coaching, particularly in healthcare. But if we focus on the skills demonstrated in formal coaching or in a coaching conversation, it appears evident that their existence in the day-to-day experience of the NHS would go a long way to improve the maternity workplace culture for staff and the experience of women.

When considering recent inquiries into maternity services, a coaching mindset is absent in the more concerning accounts of service user and staff experiences. The Report of the Morecambe Bay Investigation (2015), an investigation into the deaths of 11 babies and one mother at University of Morecambe Bay NHS Trust (Kirkup 2015), highlighted a repeated lack of empathy and compassion for women and their families. Similarly, an independent investigation into East Kent NHS Trust (Kirkup 2022) identified multiple instances of staff being shouted at, humiliated, and even experiencing racism, contributing to a '*daunting and frightening work environment*' (p. 14). In both reports, it is evident that when staff are mistreated, it rippled down to women. When you consider the recurrent concerns that women voiced in the investigations of 2015 and 2022 such as *I wasn't listened to* and *they didn't seem to care* it doesn't take a huge leap to imagine a workplace where staff are listened to and cared for and that this experience would inevitably ripple down to the experience of service users.

## 5.14  Next Steps

Some of you may already have experienced the benefits of being coached or are currently working as a coach. Others might be considering training to become a coach or are simply interested in being coached. Whatever your aspirations, there can be no doubt that if we all worked to enhance our coaching skills, we would reap the rewards by having more meaningful, thought-provoking conversations. If you're thinking about training, it's important to do some thorough research before you decide on a provider. If you're interested in being coached, consider the following:

**What do you want the focus of your coaching to be on?** If it's to develop your leadership skills, advance your career, enhance performance, or build your resilience in the workplace, you'll need to decide whether to access coaching internally through your organisation or seek an external coach.

**Internal coaching** The benefit is that it's often free of charge. However, while there may be claims that everyone can access coaching (at least in England), the reality might not be so straightforward.

**External coaching** If you wish to focus on non-work issues or prefer privacy from your manager, seeking an external coach may be the better option. Though this usually involves a cost, many coaches offer pro bono services.

**Questions to Ask When Choosing a Coach**
**Is your coach accredited?** Have they undertaken recognised training, engaged in ongoing professional development, and regularly access supervision? Beware of online adverts offering 'free' coaching qualifications—they are best avoided.

**What do the testimonials say**? Always check for feedback from previous coachees.

**Is the issue sensitive**? If it's something you'd rather not discuss with someone within your organisation, external coaching may be more appropriate. Many prospective coachees seek coaching for leadership development or career exploration, but others may need coaching for more personal or confidential matters.

While anyone can engage in coaching conversations, it's important to distinguish between a coaching conversation and a formal coaching session. Key distinctions between the two are as follows:

**Ownership of the outcome** In formal coaching, the coachee owns the outcome. The coach's role is to guide, not to direct, unless there's a risk of harm to the coachee or others. In contrast, in a coaching conversation within an organisation, such as during 1:1 meetings, the leader often holds ownership of the outcome on behalf of the organisation.

**Objectivity**  Coaches should maintain impartiality and avoid coaching individuals with whom they have a close relationship or where there might be a conflict of interest. This ensures that the coach remains neutral and focused on supporting the coachee without personal bias or investment in the outcome.

In conclusion, while coaching conversations can happen in various settings, the distinctions between a coaching conversation and formal coaching, particularly around ownership of outcomes and objectivity, are crucial. Upholding these principles ensures the effectiveness of coaching and protects both the coach and coachee from potential conflicts of interest.

## 5.15   Conclusion

If the 'golden thread' of developing a coaching mindset is woven through maternity services, it has the potential to transform workplace culture in a way that benefits staff and women. While we all possess the foundational skills to engage in coaching conversations, these skills may require fine-tuning and practice. When applied effectively, these skills will make individuals feel that they matter. They will also empower them to make better decisions and enhance their performance and resilience. The positive impact on the organisation is profound.

It is important that we disentangle the differences between coaching and sports coaching as although they share common principles, they do differ in their focus and application. Whereas sports coaching often emphasises the transfer of knowledge, akin to mentoring, coaching is focused on supporting and empowering the individual to think for themselves. This approach enables people to build self-worth, to identify their priorities, and to think for themselves. This approach enables people to build self-worth, identify their priorities, and take meaningful steps towards achieving their aspirations. Mentoring has long been established as the cornerstone of developing maternity staff, but on its own, it can have its limitations. Introducing a stronger coaching approach alongside mentoring can complement and significantly enhance its outcomes.

Coaching is powerful. It can be applied at any time—at the start of a career and at the end and everywhere in between. It will foster stronger relationships and therefore has the potential to reduce those negative behaviours that are so damaging in the work environment. It could be the 'golden thread' that unites students, staff and service users and drives positive change across maternity services.

## References

Anderson D, Anderson M (2005) Coaching that Counts. Elsevier, Oxford

Association for Coaching (n.d.-a) UK, London. https://www.associationforcoaching.com. Accessed 27 Dec 2024

Association for Coaching (n.d.-b) Vision and Objectives. In: AC Vision and Purpose. Association for Coaching. Available: https://www.associationforcoaching.com. Accessed 2 August 2024

Baron-Cohen S (2012) Zero Degrees of Empathy – A New Theory of Human Cruelty and Kindness. Penguin Books, UK

Brown B (2021) Atlas of the Heart – Mapping Meaningful Connection and the Language of Human Experience. Penguin, Random House, UK

Burt S (2019) The Art of Listening in Coaching and Mentoring. Routledge, London

Covey SR (2004) The Seven Habits of Highly Effective People: Powerful Lessons in Personal Change. Simon & Schuster, UK

Clear J (2018) Atomic Habits: An Easy and Proven Way to Build Good Habits & Break Bad Ones. Penguin, Random House, UK

Clutterbuck D (2007) Coaching the Team at Work. London, Boston.

Finnerty G, Collington V (2013) Practical coaching by mentors: student midwives' perceptions. Nurse Educ Pract. 2013 Nov;13(6): 573–7. https://doi.org/10.1016/j.nepr.2012.09.015. Epub 2012 Nov 17. PMID23164976.

Hadikin R, O'Driscoll M (2000) The Bullying Culture. Butterworth-Heinemann Publications, UK

Infant and Toddler Forum (2019) Making Every Contact Count – From Pregnancy to Preschool. https://infantandtoddlerforum.org/media/upload/pdf-downloads/ITF212_Factsheet_1_10_MECC.pdf (Accessed 18 Jan 2025)

International Coaching Federation (2025) The International Coaching Federation. https://www.coachingfederation.org.uk/ (Accessed 18 Jan 2025)

Iordanou I, Hawley R, Iordanou C (2017) Values and Ethics in Coaching. Sage Publications Ltd, London, New York

Katzenbach JR, Smith DK (1999) The Wisdom of Teams: Creating the High-Performance Organization. Harper-Business Keyworth, London

Keyworth C, Epton T, Goldthorpe J, Calam R. and Armitage JA. (2018) Are healthcare professionals delivering opportunistic behaviour change interventions? A multi-professional survey of engagement with public health policy. Implementation Science 13, Article number 122

Kirkup B (2015) The report of the Morecambe Bay investigation. The Stationary Office, Preston

Kirkup B (2022) Reading the Signals: maternity and neonatal services in East Kent – the Report of the Independent Investigation. The Stationary Office.

Kline N (2002) Time to Think, Listening to Ignite the Human Mind. Ward Lock, Cassell Illustrated, London

Lally P, Van Jaarsveld CHM, Potts HWW, Wardle J (2010) How are habits formed: Modelling habit formation in the real world. European Journal of Social Psychology 40(6):998–1009. Available: https://doi.org/10.1002/ejsp.674 (Accessed 25 Jan 2025)

Lawrence W, Black C, Tinati T, Cradock S, Begum R, Jarman M, Pease A, Margetts B, Davies J, Inskip H, Cooper C, Baird J, Barker M (2016). Making every contact count': Evaluation of the impact of an intervention to train health and social care practitioners in skills to support health behaviour change. Journal Health Psychol. 2016 Feb; 21(2):138–51. https://doi.org/10.1177/1359105314523304. Epub 2014 Apr 8. PMID 24713156: PMC4678584

McGill I, Beaty L (1992) Action Learning: A Practitioner's Guide. Kogan Page Ltd, London

NHS Leadership Academy (2025a) NHS Leadership Academy. Available: https://www.leadershipacademy.nhs.uk (Accessed 18 Jan 2025)

NHS Leadership Academy (2025b) Regional coaching and mentoring offers. Available: https://www.leadershipacademy.nhs.uk/programmes/coaching-and-mentoring/regional-coaching-and-mentoring-offers/ (Accessed 18 Jan 2025)

NHS Standard Contract (2023–24) Service Condition 8: Unmet Needs, Making Every Contact Count and Self Care. Available: https://www.england.nhs.uk/wp-content/uploads/2021/12/3-nhs-standard-contract-fl-service-conditions.pdf (Accessed 18 Jan 2025)

Nursing and Midwifery Council (NMC). Standards for pre-registration midwifery programmes (2023). Available: https://www.nmc.org.uk/globalassets/sitedocuments/standards/2024/standards-for-pre-registration-midwifery-programmes.pdf (Accessed 18 Jan 2025).

Nursing and Midwifery Council (2019) Standards for Midwives. Available: https://www.nmc.org.uk/standards/standards-for-midwives/standards-of-proficiency-for-midwives/ (Accessed 18 Jan 2025)

New South Wales (NSW) Government (2025) Get Healthy Service. Available: https://www.gethealthynsw.com.au/ (Accessed 18 Jan 2025)

O'Connor S, Cavanagh M (2013) The coaching ripple effect: The effects of development coaching on wellbeing across organisational networks. Psych Well-Being 3 (2). Available: https://doi.org/10.1186/2211-1522-3-2 (Accessed 18 Jan 2025)

Pedrick C (2021) Simplifying Coaching: How to Have More Transformational Conversations by Doing Less. McGraw Hill, Open University Press, London, New York.

Public Health England (2016) Making Every Contact Count (MECC): Consensus statement. Available: https://assets.publishing.service.gov.uk/media/5c338360e5274a65a5da03d5/Making_Every_Contact_Count_Consensus_Statement.pdf (Accessed 18 Jan 2025)

Sinclair A, Fairhurst P, Carter A, Miller L (2008) Evaluation of Coaching in the NHS. Institute for Employment Studies, England. Available: https://www.employment-studies.co.uk/system/files/resources/files/nhsi_0408.pdf (Accessed 18 Jan 2025)

Starr J (2008) Brilliant Coaching: How to be a brilliant coach in your workplace. Pearson Education Ltd, London

Starr J (2011) The Coaching Manual, The definitive guide to the process, principles and skills of personal coaching. Pearson Education Ltd, London

Starr J (2021) The Coaching Manual: Your Step-by-Step Guide to Becoming a Great Coach. Pearson Education Ltd, London

Oxford English Dictionary (2024) Oxford University Press, Oxford. Available: https://www.oed.com/search/dictionary/?scope=Entries&q=Listen (Accessed 18 Jan 2025)

Oxford English Dictionary (2025b) Oxford University Press. Oxford. Available at: https://www.oxfordlearnersdictionaries.com/definition/english/golden-thread?q=golden+thread (Accessed 28 Feb 2025)

Thomas C (2022) Coaching and mentoring skills: a complement to the professional midwifery advocate role. BJM 30 (5). Available: https://www.britishjournalofmidwifery.com/content/professional/coaching-and-mentoring-skills-a-complement-to-the-professional-midwifery-advocate-role/ (Accessed 18 Jan 2025)

Weil S (1948) Gravity and Grace. Routledge and Kegan Paul, London

Weingarten E In: From One to Many: How the Coaching Ripple Effect Transforms Individuals, Teams and Organizations. TORCH. 2023. Available: https://torch.io/blog/coaching-ripple-effect/ (Accessed 18 Jan 2025)

World Health Organisation (2021) WHO Template: Initiatives that have strengthened Nursing and Midwifery Jobs/Education/Leadership/ Service Delivery in 2021.

Whitmore J (2009) Coaching for Performance: GROWing Human Potential and Purpose. The Principles and Practice of Coaching Leadership, 4th ed. Nicholas Brealey Publishing, London, Boston

Wise K (2020) 'What is Coaching: 10 Definitions,' Available: https://karenwise.wordpress.com/2010/05/20/what-is-coaching-10-definitions/ (Accessed 17 Dec 2024)

# The Value of Schwartz Rounds in Changing Culture

**6**

Emer Kelly

## 6.1 Introduction

Schwartz Rounds can be powerful catalysts for achieving a positive maternity culture. They are confidential, reflective forums to enable both healthcare students and staff to consider the rewards and challenges of working in clinical practice (The Point of Care Foundation 2025). Reflection can provide improvements in patient care, and this can lead to staff engagement and enhancement of well-being (Lown and Manning 2010; Goodrich 2012; Wren 2014). These rounds foster psychological safety to encourage all attendees to reflect on the emotional aspects of their work. The fundamental basis for Schwartz Rounds is that compassionate care has a significant impact on women and birthing people's care experience. Furthermore, a supportive workforce is required for healthcare workers to deliver safe, compassionate care (Dasan et al. 2015). They are a non-judgemental way to provide support to all, reinforcing our values, reminding us why we chose our profession and restoring commitment to compassionate care (Lown and Manning 2010; Goodrich 2012).

## 6.2 What Are Schwartz Rounds?

Themes of stories are generated to all students and staff within the healthcare faculty of the University and students then express their interest to share a story. Each storyteller is contacted by the facilitators who discuss their story and address any questions or concerns they may have prior to the round, ensuring that they feel comfortable with sharing their story. Each round typically lasts 60 min where a group of three or four students and/or staff share a story that had a remarkable impact on

E. Kelly (✉)
University of Southampton, Southampton, United Kingdom
e-mail: E.L.Kelly@soton.ac.uk

© The Author(s), under exclusive license to Springer Nature
Switzerland AG 2025
M. O'Brien, E. Kitson-Reynolds (eds.), *Respectful Relationships in the Maternity
Service*, https://doi.org/10.1007/978-3-032-04281-1_6

them. Refreshments are provided for attendees, which contributes to all members feeling a sense of being *cared for* and *valued*. These stories are then used to create a wider deeper reflective discussion with all attendees at the round and how these stories resonate with them (Gleeson et al. 2020). All discussions are guided by facilitators who extract themes from the stories shared, enabling interpersonal connectedness (Point of Care Foundation 2025). Once the stories are shared, the Schwartz Round facilitator will seek emotive words used by the storytellers. They will make links, provide validation and reflection, and check for meaning to deepen the discussion, summarising the key themes identified. This allows for a deeper meaning and understanding of the story to be unveiled. These rounds have a snowball effect where once a story is shared, other staff members and students come forward with their own experiences.

Schwartz Rounds differ from clinical supervision as they are not about fixing problems or improving practice (Maben et al. 2018). Despite not being therapy sessions, the feedback from attendees is very positive with reports of the rounds being found to be therapeutic (Barker et al. 2016). Schwartz Rounds do not focus on the clinical aspects of care, but explore the emotional aspects, which in turn may assist staff to effectively develop their own coping mechanism (Taylor et al. 2018; The Point of Care Foundation 2025). Sharing a story often helps to achieve a deeper level of reflection and to see an experience in a different light. Stories shared are from a variety of disciplines of health professionals, which provides increased insight for students from a range of perspectives. This also enables connection, resonance and commonality when others share similar emotions, which can enhance appreciation of each other's roles (Gleeson et al. 2020). This in turn is known to improve working relationships and enhanced teamwork (Maben et al. 2018).

## 6.3    History of Schwartz Rounds and Where Do They Originate From?

Schwartz Rounds stem from Kenneth Schwartz who was a Boston-based healthcare lawyer who sadly died of lung cancer in his early 40s. During his career, he was very knowledgeable about healthcare policies and government regulations, but had less insights into the delivery of care. This delivery of care became more apparent throughout his illness when he was exposed to chemotherapy, radiation and surgery and his interactions with interprofessional teams within healthcare. Before he died, he wrote about the positive impact of receiving compassionate care, acts of kindness from the health professionals and how this made the 'unbearable bearable' (Schwartz 1995). Kenneth Schwartz authored an article in the *Boston Globe*, describing the care he received during his illness focusing on how '*small acts of kindness made the unbearable bearable*' (Schwartz 1995, p. 1). During his medical care, Schwartz observed the disparities in the way staff exhibited compassion towards him. He summed this up that intense hospital environments can 'stifle inherent compassion and humanity' (Schwartz 1995, p. 3). Moreover, this brought light to how challenging work environments can reduce the compassion displayed by health professionals and this inspired Kenneth Schwartz to reflect on how this materialises.

Schwartz Rounds were introduced to the United Kingdom in 2009 by The Point of Care Foundation and implemented in both healthcare settings and, thereafter, universities (The Point of Care Foundation 2014). The Francis Inquiry (2013) identified lack of compassion as a failing in care; (see Sect. 2.2) following on from this report, Schwartz Rounds were recommended as a way of encouraging compassionate care for both staff and women and birthing people in their care (Maben et al. 2021). Cultural change is required (Francis Inquiry 2013) to promote compassion and support for staff, which, as discussed in Chap. 3, has been shown to improve safety and patient care. For cultural change to be implemented, healthcare professionals must be invested in at undergraduate level (Pecukonis et al. 2008).

## 6.4    The Importance of Education

Education is vital to achieving culture change and implementing compassionate care and Schwartz Rounds can address this issue (Leamy et al. 2019). Fostering a compassionate workforce needs to commence when students start their undergraduate training. At the time of writing, there are 47 Higher Education Institutes (HEIs) within the United Kingdom (UK) running Schwartz Rounds for undergraduate healthcare students. The Nursing and Midwifery Council (NMC) (NMC 2018) code states that care must be compassionate, emphasising the significance of moral values for midwives providing care and those supporting student learning (NMC 2018). Schwartz Rounds provide an opportunity for all healthcare students to reflect on their experiences of clinical placements in a structured forum.

A pilot study by Stocker et al. (2018) showed that implementing Schwartz Rounds early in undergraduate programs encouraged increased awareness for both reflective practice and self-awareness of requirements needed to assist students' continuing professional development. Over 50% of students within this study demonstrated learning needs through attendance at the rounds. In the study undertaken by Maben et al. (2021), interviewees described these rounds as *'reflective learning spaces'* (Maben et al. 2021, p. 17).

Attendance at Schwartz Rounds has also been shown to increase empathy (Smith et al. 2020), resilience, teamworking and reflection skills amongst undergraduate students (Barker et al. 2016; Gishen et al. 2016). Through reflection, enhanced understanding of insight and well-being is increased, which in turn can assist in developing compassionate care within healthcare professional Interprofessional Education (IPE) and Schwartz Rounds can contribute to a positive learning experience for students. This is evident from research carried out by Abnett et al. (2022), where students acknowledged the benefits of IPE and how this deepened their understanding of other member's roles.

## 6.4.1 The Journey of a Healthcare Student

As health professionals, we often 'detach' ourselves from our work and 'control' our emotions (Pepper et al. 2012). This detachment often occurs during extreme pressures of the work environment. Withholding feelings may further reduce compassion (Walker and Mann 2016). Furthermore, Walker and Mann (2016) have described this as a *'professional armour'* (Walker and Mann 2016, p. 188). Feeling safe to share concerns and vulnerabilities within healthcare is paramount for both students and staff.

A national evaluation of Schwartz Rounds established that attendees reported a marked improvement in psychological well-being (Maben et al. 2017). Additionally, reduced stress levels and feeling less isolated with increased understanding of empathy were also reported (Lown and Manning 2010; Maben et al. 2018). Psychological safety is outlined by Edmondson (1999). It *'describes a team climate characterised by interpersonal trust and mutual respect in which people are comfortable being themselves'* (Edmondson 1999, p. 354) and is of prime importance for both student and staff well-being.

Throughout their 3-year undergraduate degree, students experience a wide range of challenges inclusive of attending to their well-being and building up coping mechanisms to enhance resilience, though more needs to be done here (NMC 2018). The difference with healthcare students is that a considerable amount of their time is spent in clinical practice. For midwifery students, 50% of their course is theory and 50% practice with students required to spend a minimum of 2300 h in practice throughout their undergraduate degree (NMC 2018).

For healthcare students, stress can be experienced from the beginning of their training, and increases further as training progresses. Core to midwifery education is learning about professional values, behaviours and acknowledgment of our own well-being (See Sect. 4.3). When we become detached from our professional values, stress increases and compassion is limited (Curtis et al. 2012). Furthermore, this may lead to burnout and absences (Maben 2013). Stress is a common reason for staff absences within healthcare in the UK (West 2019). Ultimately, if we are unable to prioritise our own well-being, then it is questionable as to how we can care for women and birthing people. Stress can impact on our ability to provide compassionate care (Mathieu 2007) and effective supportive mechanisms for students are vital to address these pressures and burnout. Schwartz Rounds have been shown to reduce these pressures that contribute to psychological stress (Dawson et al. 2021; Maben et al. 2018).

Healthcare professionals will endure uncomfortable experiences throughout their career, which can impact well-being. Midwifery students are exposed to a wide array of experiences in clinical settings, from dealing with normal birth, caring for vulnerable women and birthing people and their families, safeguarding, maternal and neonatal death. These experiences can lead to psychological exhaustion if additional support is not provided (Maben 2013). Schwartz Rounds can unite all and enable a sense of connectedness and belonging, which can encourage a compassionate culture. Reflection on the emotional aspects of working as a healthcare professional is sometimes not explored enough. For students, there are increased pressures on clinical hours, completing skills, achieving competencies and gaining knowledge. Although students are required to reflect throughout their degree, further emphasis here is required. Schwartz Rounds can close this gap and assist in developing empathetic, compassionate and resilient members of the workforce (Barker et al. 2016).

This group reflection has been proved to address a range of issues students and staff experience in clinical practice (Maben et al. 2018; Robert et al. 2017). This mutual understanding can enhance student and staff relationships, improve insights of each other's roles and reinforce effective teamwork (Maben et al. 2018). For students, observation of staff members being open with their emotional experiences can normalise these feelings as well as breaking down any hierarchy (Clancy et al. 2019).

According to Zervos and Gishen (2019), the focal point of Schwartz Rounds is about *'the humanity in healthcare'* (Zervos and Gishen 2019, p. 409). They explain that empathy is not always the focus within teachings with more attention on academic excellence and progress. It could be argued that there is limited time to incorporate this within educational settings or there is an assumption that healthcare professionals come into this caring profession with empathy. Nonetheless, empathetic care is core to midwifery education. High-quality safe care for women and birthing people requires staff to be compassionate and display empathy (Sinclair et al. 2016). Attendance at Schwartz Rounds can enhance the connection of all through sharing stories, which can reinforce compassion and empathy. Central to a compassionate workforce is for staff to feel valued, which is shown to increase levels of engagement and satisfaction (Worline and Dutton 2017).

Gishen et al. (2016), through a mixed-methods evaluation of Schwartz Rounds found that 80% of students had planned to attend future rounds and 64% of students suggested for rounds to be part of the curriculum. Students also appreciated the opportunity to reflect without it being an assigned piece of work. Similarly, Gleeson et al. (2020) explored Schwartz Rounds as a means of effective reflective practice. Students within this study also favoured this form of reflection to written. Schwartz Rounds differ from lectures and teaching of skills, as no assessment is required, presenting them as a unique safe place for all to share emotions and vulnerabilities (Taylor et al. 2018). This enables us to develop deeper insights into our vulnerabilities, develop reflective skills, being open and honest and drawing out our 'human' side. Open and honest communication can highlight to students the importance of sharing emotional challenges, which in turn can enhance communication skills and perhaps coping mechanisms (Taylor et al. 2018).

## 6.5    Benefits of Schwartz Rounds—How They Can Support Healthcare Staff and Students

Results from The National Health Service (NHS) Staff Survey 2022 identified that 44.8% of staff had felt unwell due to work-related stress in the previous 12 months and 37.4% reported their work to be emotionally exhausting (NHS Staff Survey 2022). Schwartz Rounds were included as one of five case studies after an evaluation of NHS staff well-being and that facilitating Schwartz Rounds was deemed positive and cost effective (The International Public Policy Observatory 2022).

Students and staff who attend Schwartz Rounds have reported feeling less pressure and feelings of isolation within their work environment (Maben et al. 2018). These rounds are a safe space to discuss and normalise emotions that arise from clinical practice, which can reduce burdens often placed on healthcare staff. Barker et al. (2016) obtained qualitative data from a focus group which identified students value these rounds as they link to well-being, stress, and burnout with recommendations for normalising emotions. Shared storytelling can initiate self-reflection and prompt attendees to perhaps reconsider and recognise their own feelings as normal (McCarthy et al. 2021; Allen et al. 2020).

Shared experiences through storytelling encourage open communication and unite and connect all involved. This open communication highlights the value of discussing our concerns and vulnerabilities. Acknowledgement and resonating with how others feel can help normalise one's own feelings. (McCarthy et al. 2021). Compassionate care and improved well-being are likely to be accomplished during these rounds (George 2016; Maben 2013). Clancy et al. (2019) conducted interpretative phenomenological analysis of interviews with Schwartz Round attenders and three themes were identified.

1. Students can question if it is safe to share within Schwartz Rounds.
2. Students reporting not feeling alone with experiences and emotions.
3. Having space and time to discuss professional cultures.

The third point, having time to discuss professional cultures, is not always possible (Clancy et al. 2019). This connection can also enable a better understanding of different team member's roles which leads to effective teamworking.

Hierarchies are broken down during rounds and this was evident from my own experience of sharing a story. It was a very meaningful experience to see the connection of all members within the round. During these rounds, we leave our professional identity at the door and come together as humans discussing the emotive aspects of our work. This enhances staff engagement, role-modelling behaviours and exploring vulnerabilities within a safe space (Maben et al. 2017). Sharing a story and role-modelling compassionate care can reignite and increase compassion amongst those listening.

The following case study is a true description of the author's first experience of attending a Schwartz Round and in the role of a storyteller. The theme for the Schwartz Rounds on this day was 'A person I will always remember'. This took the author back to a patient she had cared for in Intensive Care Unit (ICU) during the COVID pandemic in 2020. I shared this story for the first time 4 years after the experience. As many health professionals who worked during this time, it really did feel like our NHS was falling to pieces and there appeared to be no solutions to address this.

> **Box 6.1 Vignette—Sharing a Story During a Schwartz Round**
>
> Within both my nursing and midwifery career, I have gained lots of experience within a wide range of clinical settings. However, I remember feeling apprehensive due to the alarming death rates and fear of the unknown. We put on our masks and went to work like soldiers on a battlefield. The kindness and compassion from colleagues at the time were the only saving grace that enabled me to get out of bed in the morning and face the dreaded ward with the death rate continuing to rise.
>
> I was allocated to care for a 60-year-old man who had been in ICU for 5 weeks. Prior to his hospital admission, he was fit and healthy. He had been on a ventilator and now extubated and receiving continuous positive airway pressure (CPAP). I was informed that this patient/service user was challenging and aggressive towards staff. When I first met this patient, he looked frustrated and withdrawn. He was slumped in the bed and biting his lip, and his facial expression reminded me of my own Dad whom I had lost prior to COVID. It took me a long time to build a trusting relationship with this patient. In the beginning, he would swear at me and tell me to go home. I saw this behaviour as fear and was determined for him to engage with me. He was not able to transfer to a commode so was using a bedpan. I could see he was also carrying the emotional burden of shame and embarrassment. I found these episodes of care very difficult and sometimes biting my own lip to stop myself from crying. I found the personal protective equipment (PPE) could hide a multitude of emotions. I was very conscious that it was not about me but the care that I was providing for this patient. However, I felt that by displaying some emotion, it enabled me to be more 'human'.
>
> After 4 weeks of caring for this patient, I felt that his demeanour had changed and he became more personable and further engaged with me. I cared for this patient for 3 months and am delighted to say I was on shift when he was discharged home.

Sometimes, we mask our feelings as health professionals and sharing this story taught me how it was ok to share our vulnerabilities. Being able to share my vulnerabilities also broke down any hierarchies and validation from attendees in the room helped me to identify my feelings as 'normal'.

I have experienced both maternal and neonatal deaths and cared for dying patients in my nursing career, but nothing prepared me for the exhaustion and grim reality of working in ICU during COVID. We are thought to be resilient in healthcare, but I feel that by 'letting down my guard' enabled me to display more empathy and compassion. I also feel that by displaying some emotion, it strengthened my relationship with this patient.

During this experience, I discussed that being able to be 'emotional' during this time enabled me to be more compassionate. Bearing in mind, my red swollen eyes were not always visible under my goggles and visor. However, to me, this was my 'professional armour' and without this, I am unsure if I would have been able to provide compassionate care whilst keeping my emotions locked away. Withholding my emotions may have been counterproductive and inhibit my ability to provide compassionate care. I found this experience very cathartic and healing to 'normalise' my emotions. Understanding differing viewpoints and feeling a sense of belonging enhanced the connectedness within the room.

> **Box 6.2 Exercise—Recognising When We Are Emotionally Vulnerable**
> Can you remember withholding emotions when caring for a patient/woman or birthing person and would you do anything differently if you were to be in this situation again?
>
> Do you feel as health professionals there is stigma associated with exposing our vulnerabilities?
>
> Think about an experience where you required psychological support to assist you within your role and how this may have made a difference.

Through role modelling, students can feel more comfortable to engage and not only do you learn about yourself but through others' perspectives.

Smith et al. (2020), through their evaluation of pilot Schwartz Round survey feedback, identified appreciation for hearing other experiences and found that this generated empathy. Storytelling from senior members of staff not only breaks down any hierarchies but can enable all to see and hear experiences from a wide range of perspectives. This was evident from Clancy et al.'s (2019) research, where students reported feeling *'safe'* and a unique opportunity to reflect on professional cultures as well as decreasing interprofessional boundaries. In addition, students also valued hearing the *'more human'* side from senior members of staff (Gishen et al. 2016). Schwartz Rounds can provide an excellent role-modelling experience for students which enhances the connection of all involved.

## 6.6 Stories Are Powerful to Enhance Shared Understanding

Here are some examples of story topics shared at Schwartz Rounds: 'The Person in the Professional', 'A patient/experience I will never forget', 'The day I made a difference' and 'In at the deep end'. There is the potential for these topics to generate interest through a broad range of perspectives.

The stories shared identify vulnerabilities, dealing with the unknown, having faith and hope and allow for deep reflection. The rounds focus on our personal feelings and the impact this has on us. They are about our emotional reactions to clinical situations and how we react personally to these (Maben et al. 2017). Within this safe space, validating and normalising feelings can empower individuals, which in turn can enhance compassionate care (George 2016). From my experience as a facilitator, these rounds enable us to process stories on a deeper level. The environment is safe, and everybody is welcomed. The level of emotion is palpable and a very meaningful experience. Stories are reflective and powerful and can reveal insights into a person's personality and way of life (Haigh and Hardy 2011). Our lives are a collection of stories. Every healthcare worker has a story to share. As human beings, we are *'built to absorb, interpret, and respond to stories'* (Charon 2001, p. 1897).

An old saying comes to mind: *'A problem shared is a problem halved'*. This is likely to be replicated with sharing a story that had an impact on us emotionally. Kirkpatrick et al. (1997) describe storytelling as *'…the individual account of an event to create a memorable picture in the mind of the listener'* (Kirkpatrick et al. 1997 p. 38). Stories within healthcare can promote professional identity and bring a group closer together, enhancing safe practice and patient care (Kirkpatrick et al. 1997; Roberts 2000; Gaydos 2005; Hardy 2007; Charon 2009; Haigh and Hardy 2011). Storytelling within Schwartz Rounds are focused on human experience and not the professional experience. This safe space allows for deep reflection and further understanding of our beliefs. According to East et al. (2010), stories 'convey values and emotions and can reveal the differences and similarities between people's experiences' (East et al. 2010, p. 17). When we share stories, we develop understanding and empathy which can encourage an emotional connection and acceptance (Hayes et al. 2012). Appreciation of a colleague's experience through storytelling provides insights into their values, beliefs, relationships, expectations and responsibilities (Sakalys 2003). Storytelling has been shown to have a therapeutic effect on the well-being of both the storyteller and the listeners.

Sharing a story is known to stimulate the cortical, parietal, subcortical and frontal portions of the brain, contributing to enhanced recollection of events discussed (Wendy and Suzuki 2018). This is likely to benefit students with different learning needs and differs substantially from the traditional lecture format, which may not be effective for all students. Much research has been written about narrative pedagogy (Diekelmann 2001) and the powerful impact this has on healthcare students with an alternative means of developing reflective and critical thinking skills (Andrews et al. 2001; Ironside 2015). Furthermore, this can enhance staff relationships and reducing isolation, creating a positive work culture. Revealing the person behind the profession and breaking down hierarchies can enhance staff engagement, increase staff morale, which in turn can foster a psychologically safe workplace (Maben et al. 2018). Storytellers are encouraged to share their feelings, experiences and perceptions without judgement. Sharing experiences in a safe environment can be therapeutic and enable students to release stress/anxiety that may have been bottled up. This in turn can create deep reflection and self-awareness and enable individuals to be empowered. In addition, this is an opportunity to understand and renew knowledge base and equip with skills to respond to the unknown (Fischer 2018).

Listening to shared stories is to a degree therapeutic and encourages empathy and connection (Hibbin 2016; Yoder-Wise and Kowalski 2003). Storytelling can inspire others to come forward and share their experience, which can lead to a culture of understanding and compassion. Lipsey et al. (2020) identified that storytelling can potentially reduce fears for others who had similar experiences, and this is more relatable for students compared to taught lessons (Lipsey et al. 2020). This is an opportunity to connect and be 'human' and can also cultivate resilience. Psychological literature dating back to the 90s also supports this and highlights that storytelling offers both authentication and validation (White and Epston 1990).

Validation during these rounds is pivotal for all involved. Validation is demonstrating understanding of that person's experience without judgement (Koerner 2012; Koerner and Linehan 2003). Communication with increased levels of validation is linked to increased understanding and fulfilment, which enable trust and engagement (Fruzzetti and Worrall 2010).

## 6.7 Organisational Benefits of Schwartz Rounds

Support, trust and respect are integral for all team members within their workplace. This open culture enables compassionate care to thrive and in turn can positively influence organisational culture (Maben et al. 2018). Schwartz Rounds not only empower staff but also realign them with their passion for working within healthcare, which can lead to compassionate leadership. Compassionate leadership allows for an effective, more engaged team, which in turn leads to safe high-quality care (West 2021). This is clearly the missing part of the puzzle that remains within our NHS today. This detachment and passion for the caring role was first brought to light by the Francis Report (Francis Inquiry 2013). This report showed that staff lacked compassion for the patients in their care. Sir Francis concluded that this insensitive behaviour was a result from the toxic workplace culture. Fundamentally, this toxic culture was because of ineffective teamwork and leadership. Sir Francis contended that a change in culture was required and would only be achieved if compassionate partnership of the workforce was adopted. Furthermore, organisational culture has been attributed to burnout in comparison to patient care or individual components (Watts et al. 2013; Green et al. 2014). Schwartz Rounds enables all to reconnect and assess our moral principles and values. Open communication provides transparency and a safe and trusting environment, which enhances effective teamwork and compassionate care (McCarthy et al. 2021). Schwartz Rounds have been compared to

> a space for dialogue between participants that is safe, secure, and supportive, that stands in between the formal areas of practice. (Moje et al. 2004, p. 43)

## 6.8    Conclusion

Investing in and developing our future NHS workforce are paramount and nursing, midwifery and medical professional bodies have identified that further steps are required to address resilience within their training (GMC 2015; NMC 2017). Pressures are experienced from the get-go of training and as commitments increase, so do pressures and this has been shown to have a reduction in the levels of empathy displayed, especially when support is absent (Burks and Kobus 2012; Park et al. 2015). Professional norms and social identity can be set aside and focus on meeting NHS-driven targets. Students may feel overwhelmed, and this can create conflicts in their beliefs and what is required to achieve compassionate care. Introducing Schwartz Rounds at the beginning of their training is anticipated to offer students a safe and confidential forum to reflect and in turn influence cultural change (Barker et al. 2016). IPE enables shared communication which in turn enhances interprofessional working (Bridges et al. 2011). Student feedback echoes this and shows appreciation of how interprofessional learning can enhance their understanding of each other's roles (Abnett et al. 2022).

Even though there is no quick-fix solution to our current NHS workforce issues and culture, Schwartz Rounds can positively address this, and research does demonstrate that psychological well-being of staff who attended these rounds significantly improved in comparison to non-attendees (Maben et al. 2018). The rounds are safe and unique and open to all healthcare professionals, both in training and qualified. They are highly rated by those who attend and only focus on the emotional aspects of our work, abstaining from the analytical tasks of providing answers or solutions. Maben et al. (2021) elaborate on Wren's (2014) description of Schwartz Rounds as counter-cultural, proposing that they 'shift an organisation and its workers away from their default position of urgent action, reaction and problem solving to an hour of stillness and slowness'. This characterisation sums up the *uniqueness* of Schwartz Rounds and why this connection between all involved is crucial. Schwartz Rounds most definitely feel like an escape from the hustle and bustle of clinical practice and valuable time to explore and reflect on our emotional burdens.

As mentioned earlier, rounds also promote a connection through sharing stories with the focus on increasing empathy in providing compassionate care (Goodrich 2011; Maben et al. 2017; Reed et al. 2015). This focus on staff well-being may well reduce stress as well as the likelihood of burnout (Maben et al. 2017). Given the predicted shortages in the healthcare workforce, it is estimated  to be up to ten million by 2030 (WHO 2022). Much research has been carried out to evaluate the effectiveness of Schwartz Rounds and the findings certainly demonstrate that both students and staff value this safe space. Students appreciate listening to other experiences and emotions and reported a sense of feeling "…like we were fellow humans with stories rather than students" (Stocker et al. 2018, p. 3). All the studies included demonstrate the positive influence Schwartz Rounds have on both our healthcare staff and students

At the time of writing, Schwartz Rounds have been running for over a year at the author's university. They are facilitated monthly for our university students.

Attendance at the rounds is voluntary, so both students and staff can make this informed decision. The facilitators of the rounds are lecturers from different disciplines within the Health Sciences Faculty who have been provided with training and support. This training and support is ongoing and regular reflection and feedback is shared with other Higher Education Institutes (HEIs). Introductions at each round includes discussion of what to expect and emotional context. Facilitators spend time with each storyteller discussing their story and establishing the emotions they feel about their experience. Facilitators then have the role in debriefing storytellers after each round. This is an opportunity to check in with each storyteller, identify how they felt the round went and how they are feeling now.

## References

Abnett H, Tuckwell R, Evans L (2022) Early introduction of the multi-disciplinary team through student Schwartz Rounds: a mixed methodology study. BMC Med Educ. 22: 523. Available: https://doi.org/10.1186/s12909-022-03549-7 (Accessed 18 Jan 2025)

Allen D, Spencer, G, McEwan K. Catarino F. Evans R., Crooks S, Gilbert P (2020) The Schwartz Centre Rounds: Supporting mental health workers with the emotional impact of their work. Int. J Mental Health Nurs. 29 (5) 942–952.

Andrews C A, Ironside PM, Nosek C, Sims SL, Swenson MM, Yeomans C, Young PK, Diekelmann N (2001) Enacting narrative pedagogy. The lived experiences of students and teachers. Nurs. Health Care Perspect. 22 (5) 252–259.

Barker R, Cornwell J, Gishen F (2016) Introducing compassion into the education of health care professionals; can Schwartz Rounds help? J Comp Health Care. 3:3. Available: https://doi.org/10.1186/s40639-016-0020-0 (Accessed 18 Jan 2025)

Bridges D, Davidson R, Soule Odegard P, Maki, I, Tomkowiak J (2011) Interprofessional collaboration: Three best practice models of interprofessional education. M Educ Online, 16(1). Available: https://www.tandfonline.com/doi/full/10.3402/meo.v16i0.6035 (Accessed 18 Jan 2025)

Burks D, Kobus A (2012) The legacy of altruism in health care: The promotion of empathy, prosociality and humanism. Med Educ. 46(3), 317–325. Available: https://pubmed.ncbi.nlm.nih.gov/22324531/ (Accessed 18 Jan 2025)

Charon R (2009) Narrative medicine as witness for the self-telling body. J App Comm Res 37 (2):118–131.

Charon R (2001) Narrative Medicine: A Model for Empathy, Reflection, Profession, and Trust. JAMA, 286 (15):1897–1902. Available: https://jamanetwork.com/journals/jama/fullarticle/194300 (Accessed 18 Jan 2025)

Clancy D, Mitchell A, Smart C (2019) A qualitative exploration of the experiences of students attending interprofessional Schwartz Rounds in a University context. J Interprof Care. 1–10. Available: https://doi.org/10.1080/13561820.2019.1692797 (Accessed 18 Jan 2025)

Curtis K, Horton K, Smith P (2012) Student nurse socialisation in compassionate practice: A Grounded Theory study. Nurse Educ Today. 32: 790–5. Available: https://doi.org/10.1016/j.nedt.2012.04.012 (Accessed 18 Jan 2025)

Dasan S, Gohil P, Cornelius V, Taylor C (2015) Prevalence, causes and consequences of compassion satisfaction and compassion fatigue in emergency care: A mixed-methods study of UK NHS Consultants. Em Med J. 32:588–94.

Dawson J, McCarthy I, Taylor C, Hildenbrand K, Leamy M, Reynolds E, Maben J (2021) Effectiveness of a group intervention to reduce the psychological distress of healthcare staff: a pre-post quasi-experimental evaluation. BMC Health Serv Res. 2021; 21:392. Available: https://doi.org/10.1186/s12913-021-06413-4 (Accessed 25 Jan 2025)

Diekelmann N (2001) "Narrative Pedagogy: Heideggerian Hermeneutical Analyses of Lived Experiences of Students, Teachers, and Clinicians." ANS. Adv in Nurs Science **23** (3): 53–71. pmid: 11225050. Available: https://pubmed.ncbi.nlm.nih.gov/11225050/ (Accessed 4 Feb 2025)

East L, Jackson D, O'Brien L, Peters K (2010) Storytelling: an approach that can help to develop resilience. Nurse Res, 17(3):17–25. Available: https://www.westernsydney.edu.au/__data/assets/pdf_file/0019/132715/Storytelling.pdf (Accessed 4 Feb 2025)

Edmondson A (1999) Psychological safety and learning behaviour in work teams in administrative science quarterly. Adm Sci Q. 44(2):350–83. Available: https://journals.sagepub.com/doi/10.2307/2666999 (Accessed 4 Feb 2025)

Fischer JM, (2018) Near-Death Experiences: The Stories They Tell. J. Ethics. 22:97–112.

Francis R (2013) Report of the Mid Staffordshire NHS Foundation Trust Public Inquiry. Available from: https://www.gov.uk/government/publications/report-of-the-mid-staffordshire-nhs-foundation-trust-public-inquiry (Accessed 4 Feb 2025)

Fruzzetti AE, Worrall JM (2010) Accurate expression and validation: a transactional model for understanding individual and relationship distress. In: Sullivan K, Davila J, eds. Oxford: Oxford University Press. Support processes in intimate relationships.

Gaydos LH (2005) Understanding personal narratives: an approach to practice, J Adv Nursing, 49 (3):254–259.

George M (2016) Stress in NHS staff triggers defensive inward-focussing and an associated loss of connection with colleagues: This is reversed by Schwartz Rounds. J Comp Health Care, 3(9). Available: https://doi.org/10.1186/s40639-016-0025-8 (Accessed 4 Feb 2025)

Gishen F, Whitman S, Gill D, Barker R, Walker S (2016) Schwartz Centre Rounds: a new initiative in the undergraduate curriculum – what do medical students think? Med Educ 16: 246–252. Available: https://bmcmededuc.biomedcentral.com/articles/10.1186/s12909-016-0762-6 (Accessed 4 Feb 2025)

Gleeson D, Arwyn-Jones J, Awan M, White I, Halse O (2020) Medical Student Schwartz Rounds: A Powerful Medium for Medical Student Reflective Practice. Adv Med Educ Pract. 11: 775–80. Available: https://doi.org/10.2147/AMEP.S273181 (Accessed 4 Feb 2025)

GMC (2015) Promoting excellence: Standards for medical education and training. Retrieved from Available: http://www.gmc-uk.org/education/standards.asp (Accessed 4 Feb 2025)

Goodrich J (2012) Supporting hospital staff to provide compassionate care: do Schwartz center rounds work in English hospitals? J R Soc Med. 105(3): 117–22. Available: https://doi.org/10.1258/jrsm.2011.110183 (Accessed 4 Feb 2025)

Goodrich J (2011) Schwartz Center Rounds: Evaluation of the UK pilots. London, UK: The Kings Fund.

Green AE. Albanse B, Shapior NM, Aarons GA The roles of individual and organizational factors in burnout among community- based mental health service providers. Psych Services. 2014; 11:41–9.

Haigh C, Hardy P (2011) Tell me a story—A conceptual exploration of storytelling in healthcare education. Nurse Educ Today. 31, 408–411.

Hardy P (2007) An investigation into the application of the Patient Voices digital stories in healthcare education: quality of learning, policy impact and practice-based value. Belfast: University of Ulster.

Hayes, L.J., O'Brien-Pallas, L., Duffield, C., Shamian, J., Buchan, J., Hughes, F., Laschinger, H.K.S., North, N. (2012). Nurse turnover: A literature review—An update. Int. J. Nurs. Stud. 49, 887–905.

Hibbin R (2016) The psychosocial benefits of oral storytelling in school: developing identity and empathy through narrative. Past Care in Educ. 218–231.

Ironside PM (2015) "Narrative Pedagogy: Transforming Nursing Education Through 15 Years of Research in Nursing Education." Nurs Educ Persp 36(2): 83–88. https://doi.org/10.5480/13-1102. pmid: 29194131. Available: https://journals.lww.com/neponline/abstract/2015/03000/narrative_pedagogy__transforming_nursing_education.4.aspx (Accessed 4 Feb 2025)

Kirkpatrick MK, Ford S, Costelloe BP (1997) Storytelling: an approach to client-centred care, Nurse Educ. 22 (2), 38–40.

Koerner K, Linehan MM Validation principles and strategies. In: O'Donohue WT, Fisher JE, Hayes SC, eds. Cognitive behaviour therapy. Hoboken: John Wiley & Sons, 2003. pp. 456–462.

Koerner K (2012) Doing dialectical behaviour therapy: a practical guide. New York, The Guilford Press.

Leamy M, Reynolds E, Robert G, Taylor C., Maben J (2019) The origins and implementation of an intervention to support healthcare staff to deliver compassionate care: exploring fidelity and adaptation in the transfer of Schwartz Center Rounds from the United States to the United Kingdom. BMC Health Serv Res. 19(1):457. Available: https://doi.org/10.1186/s12913-019-4311-y (Accessed 4 Feb 2025)

Lipsey AF, Waterman AD, Wood EH, Balliet W (2020) Evaluation of first-person storytelling on changing health-related attitudes, knowledge, behaviours, and outcomes: A scoping review. Patient Educ. Couns. 103, 1922–1934.

Lown BA, Manning CF (2010). The Schwartz center rounds: evaluation of an interdisciplinary approach to enhancing patient-centered communication, teamwork, and provider support. Acad Med. 85(6):1073–81. Available: https://doi.org/10.1097/ACM.0b013e3181dbf741 (Accessed 4 Feb 2025)

Maben J, Taylor C, Dawson J, Leamy M, McCarthy I, Reynolds E, Ross S, Shuldham C, Burnett L, Foot C (2018) A realist informed mixed-methods evaluation of Schwartz Center Rounds in England. Health Serv Del Res. 37(No. 6) National Institute of Health Research.

Maben J (2013) Support staff to support patients. Health Serv J 123(6371):20. p. 2.12. file:///Users/margaretobrien/Downloads/Maben-Supportstafftosupportpatients.HSJFINAL.pdf (Accessed August 2024)

Maben J, Taylor C, Dawson J, Leamy M, McCarthy I, Reynolds E, Foot C (2017) A realist informed mixed methods evaluation of Schwartz Center Rounds® in England. Available from: https://njl-admin.nihr.ac.uk/document/download/2011408 (Accessed 4 Feb 2025)

Maben J, Taylor C, Reynolds E, McCarthy I, Leamy M (2021) Realist evaluation of Schwartz Rounds for enhancing the delivery of compassionate healthcare: understanding how they work, for whom, and in what contexts. BMC Health Serv. Res. 21 (709).

Mathieu F (2007) Running on empty: Compassion fatigue in health professionals. Rehab Comm Care Med. 4:1–7.

McCarthy I, Taylor C, Leamy M, Reynolds E, Maben J (2021) 'We needed to talk about it': the experience of sharing the emotional impact of health care work as a panellist in Schwartz center rounds® in the UK. J Health Services Res Policy. 26(1):20–7. Available: https://journals.sagepub.com/doi/pdf/10.1177/1355819620925512 (Accessed 4 Feb 2025)

Moje EB, Ciechanowski K.M, Kramer K, Ellis L, Carrillo R, Collazo T (2004) Working toward third space in content area literacy: an examination of every day funds of knowledge and discourse. Read Res Q. 39(1):38–70. Available: https://ila.onlinelibrary.wiley.com/doi/abs/10.1598/RRQ.39.1.4 (Accessed 4 Feb 2025)

NHS Staff Survey (2022). Available at: https://www.nhsstaffsurveys.com/results/national-results/ (Accessed 4 Feb 2025)

NMC (2017) Standards of proficiency for registered nurses. Available: https://www.nmc.org.uk/globalassets/sitedocuments/education-standards/future-nurse-proficiencies.pdf (Accessed 4 Feb 2025)

NMC (2018) The code: Professional standards of practice and behaviour for nurses, midwives and nursing associates. Available: https://www.nmc.org.uk/standards/code/ (Accessed 4 Feb 2025)

Park K, Kim D, Kim S, Yi Y, Jeong J, Chae J, Roh H (2015) The relationships between empathy, stress and social support among medical students. Inter J Med Educ. 6, 103–108. doi:https://doi.org/10.5116/ijme.55e6.0d44.

Pecukonis E, Doyle O, Bliss D (2008) Reducing barriers to interprofessional training: Promoting interprofessional cultural competence. Journal of Interprofessional Care, 22(4), 417–428. Available: https://www.tandfonline.com/doi/full/10.1080/13561820802190442 (Accessed 4 Feb 2025)

Pepper JR, Jaggar SI, Mason MJ, Finney SJ, Dusmet M (2012) Schwartz Rounds: reviving compassion in modern healthcare. J R Soc Med 105:94 –5.

The Point of Care Foundation (2025) Schwartz Rounds. Available: http://www.pointofcarefoundation.org.uk/our-work/Schwartz-rounds/ (Accessed 4 Feb 2025)

Reed E, Cullen A, Gannon C, Knight A, Todd J (2015) Use of Schwartz Centre Rounds in a UK hospice: Findings from a longitudinal evaluation. Journal of Interprofessional Care, 29(4), 365–366. Available: https://www.tandfonline.com/doi/full/10.3109/13561820.2014.983594 (Accessed 4 Feb 2025)

Robert G, Philippou J, Leamy M, Reynolds E, Ross S, Bennett L, Taylor C, Shuldham C, Maben J (2017) Exploring the adoption of Schwartz Center Rounds as an organisational innovation to improve staff well-being in England, 2009–2015. BMJ Open. Available: https://pubmed.ncbi.nlm.nih.gov/28057662/ (Accessed 4 Feb 2025)

Roberts GA (2000) Narrative and severe mental illness: what place do stories have in an evidence-based world, Advances in Psychiatric Treatment, 6, 432–441.

Sakalys JA (2003) Restoring the Patient's Voice: The Therapeutics of Illness Narratives. J. Holist. Nurs. 21, 228–241.

Schwartz K (1995) A Patient's Story. Boston: Boston Globe Magazine. Available: https://www.bostonglobe.com/magazine/1995/07/16/patient-story/q8ihHg8LfyinPA25Tg5JRN/story.html (Accessed 4 Feb 2025)

Sinclair S, Beamer K, Hack TF, McClement S, Raffin BS, Chochinov HM, Hagen NA (2016) Sympathy, empathy, and compassion: a grounded theory study of palliative care patients' understandings, experiences, and preferences. Palliat Med. 31(5):437–47.

Smith J, Stewart MG, Foggin E, Mathews S, Harris J, Thomas P, Cooney A, Stocker CJ (2020) Assessing the benefits and usefulness of Schwartz Centre Rounds in second-year medical students using clinical educator-facilitated group work session: not just "a facilitated moan" BMC Med Educ. 20: 271. Available: https://doi.org/10.1186/s12909-020-02199-x (Accessed 4 Feb 2025)

Stocker C, Cooney A, Thomas P, Kumaravel B, Langlands K, Hearn J (2018) Schwartz Rounds in undergraduate medical education facilitates active reflection and individual identification of learning need [version 1]. MedEdPublish **7**:230. Available: https://pubmed.ncbi.nlm.nih.gov/38089201/ (Accessed 4 Feb 2025)

Taylor C, Xyrichis A, Leamy M, Reynolds E, Maben J (2018) Can Schwartz Center Rounds support healthcare staff with emotional challenges at work, and how do they compare to other interventions aimed at providing similar support? A systematic review and scoping review. BMJ Open 8(10):e024254.

The International Public Policy Observatory (2022) Rapid Evidence Review and Economic Analysis: NHS Staff Wellbeing and Mental Health 2022. Available: https://theippo.co.uk/rapid-evidence-review-economic-analysis-nhs-staff-wellbeing-and-poor-mental-health/ (Accessed 4 Feb 2025)

The Point of Care Foundation (2014) Setting up and running Schwartz Center Rounds: a practical handbook. London: The Point of Care Foundation.

Walker M, Mann RA (2016) Exploration of mindfulness in relation to compassion, empathy and reflection within nursing education. Nurse Education Today, 40. pp. 188–190. Available: https://pubmed.ncbi.nlm.nih.gov/27125171/ (Accessed 4 Feb 2025)

Watts J, Robertson N, Winter R, Leeson D (2013) Evaluation of organisational culture and nurse burnout. Nursing Management. 20:24–9.

Wendy A, Suzuki M I (2018) Dialogues: The Science and Power of Storytelling. Journal of Neuroscience, 9468–9470.

West M (2019) The NHS crisis of caring for staff: what do we need to do? London: King's Fund. Available: https://www.kingsfund.org.uk/insight-and-analysis/blogs/nhs-crisis-caring-staff (Accessed 4 Feb 2025)

West MA (2021) Compassionate Leadership: Sustaining Wisdom, Humanity and Presence in Health and Social Care. London: Swirling Leaf Press.

White M, Epston D (1990) Narrative means to therapeutic ends. New York: W.W Norton & Company.

World Health Organization (2022) Working for Health 2022–2030 Action Plan. Geneva: World Health Organization. Available: https://www.who.int/publications/i/item/9789240063341 (Accessed 4 Feb 2025)

Worline MC, Dutton JE (2017) Awakening compassion at work: the quiet power that elevates people and organizations. New York City: McGraw Elevation.

Wren B (2014) Schwartz Rounds: an intervention with potential to simultaneously improve staff experience and organisational culture (Special issue of the British Psychological Society clinical psychology forum on the Francis report). Clin Psychol Forum 263:225. Available: https://pmc.ncbi.nlm.nih.gov/articles/PMC6196967/ (Accessed 4 Feb 2025)

Yoder-Wise PS, Kowalski K (2003) The power of storytelling. Volume 51, (Issue 1), 37–42.

Zervos M, Gishen F (2019) Reflecting on a career not yet lived: student Schwartz Rounds. Clin Teach. 16:409–411. Available: https://pubmed.ncbi.nlm.nih.gov/31397110/ (Accessed 4 Feb)

# Compassionate Leadership in Maternity and Neonatal Services

**7**

Maggie O'Brien

## 7.1 Introduction

This chapter draws together different perspectives to present a definition of compassionate leadership, visualising it through a range of different lenses. First, it asks what you consider compassionate leadership to be, then it discusses what we think it is and, finally, it draws together the views of leaders of maternity services who have successfully implemented culture change within their organisations. All leaders identified elements of compassionate leadership as crucial to culture change and as such it is one of the most essential 'golden threads of change' (OED 2025) (see Sect 1.5).

> Leaders need the courage to move away from traditional hierarchical leadership approaches, towards a compassionate leadership approach. It requires a sustained shift in mindset and behaviours of people working in health and care to deliver and sustain this culture change. For the sake of patients, service users, staff and communities, such sustained courage and commitment is essential. (West and Bailey 2022)

You may be asking if this chapter is for you because you do not consider yourself a leader; the answer to this is given by Smith (2021, p. 135); 'We don't necessarily need to be in a senior position to be a leader. Everyone can be a leader, championing, advocating and promoting some type of maternity care'. Leadership is potentially demonstrated by all in an organisation, not only those formally identified as leaders (West 2021). By engaging in the reflective exercises throughout the book, some readers will go on an emotional journey of self-discovery using personal experiences, and it should be seen as a strength to reach for support in safe spaces. As Brenee Brown asserts, 'A leader, first and foremost, is a human. Only when we

M. O'Brien (✉)
University of Southampton, Southampton, United Kingdom

Royal College of Midwives RCMF (Hons), London, United Kingdom
e-mail: Mahues935@gmail.com

© The Author(s), under exclusive license to Springer Nature
Switzerland AG 2025
M. O'Brien, E. Kitson-Reynolds (eds.), *Respectful Relationships in the Maternity Service*, https://doi.org/10.1007/978-3-032-04281-1_7

have the strength to show our vulnerability can we truly lead' (Brown 2025). The sea change that is required to change our cultures will not be achieved unless you are courageous and honest in your self-reflection.

## 7.2 What Is Compassionate Leadership?

The compassionate leadership approach has been developed mainly through the work and research of Professor Michael West. *What is Compassionate Leadership* (West and Bailey 2022) is a comprehensive explanation of compassionate leadership available via The King's Fund website (The Kings Fund 2025). West (2021), West et al. 2017), West and Chowla (2017), and West and Bailey (2022) consider compassionate leadership from a National Health Service (NHS)-wide perspective; it is important that we also consider what compassionate leadership is through a maternity and neonatal service lens, in particular, how it impacts on maternity staff, midwifery practice and women and birthing people.

### 7.2.1 What Do You Think Compassionate Leadership Is?

Before reading any more of this chapter, please complete the Exercise in Box 7.1; this exercise asks what you think compassionate leadership is; at the end of the chapter, we will ask if that view has changed. You may wish to explore The King's Fund website (The King's Fund 2025) and/or the NHS Leadership Academy (NHS Leadership Academy 2025) that NHS employees are encouraged to engage with.

**Box 7.1 Exercise: What Do You Think Compassionate Leadership Is?**
Please answer the following two questions:

What do you think compassionate leadership is?
What do you think compassionate leadership looks like in midwifery practice?

### 7.2.2 What We Think Compassionate Leadership Looks Like

So, what do we think compassionate leadership is and what does it look like? The theory of compassion is previously described as consisting of four elements (see Sect 2.9): *attending, understanding, empathising* and *helping* (West and Bailey 2022; West 2021, p. 3; West et al. 2017; West and Chowla 2017). Compassionate leadership involves these same four elements of compassion that are '*understood and applied in the context of leading others*' (West 2021, p. 3). West (2021) cites Lilius et al. (2011) and Worline and Boik (2006) in stating that compassionate leadership is particularly relevant in healthcare because health professionals inherently want to provide high-quality care; therefore, when leaders demonstrate compassion, they are providing support in a way that is consistent with the core values of themselves and their staff. They are also providing role modelling that encourages staff to respond compassionately in the face of suffering (West 2021). The Royal College of Midwives (RCM) (RCM 2021) uses West's (2021) definition of compassionate leadership as applying leadership principles to the four elements of attending, understanding, empathising and helping. The interpretation applied by the RCM (2021) is as follows:

*Attending*: Being present with and listening, noticing and inquiring about suffering or distress, and challenging approaches oriented to blame and punishment.
*Understanding*: It is appraising difficult situations to reach a measured understanding, ideally through open dialogue. This is grounded in the assumption that others are good, capable and worthy of value. It involves withholding blame by focusing on learning.
*Empathising*: Being able to feel the distress or frustration of those we lead without being overwhelmed by this emotion and therefore unable to help. This involves listening without needing to solve or intervene.
*Helping*: Taking thoughtful and intelligent action to help those we lead, focusing on what is most useful for them. Compassionate leadership does not involve compromising our commitment to good performance management, having difficult conversations, making radical changes or being able to challenge the status quo.

There are misconceptions within the workplace regarding what compassionate leadership is, one being that a compassionate leader is weak and unable to challenge the status quo to make radical changes. Kaufman (2023) states that 'compassion can sometimes be misconstrued as a weakness by other members of the team who don't understand its purpose or value', but goes on to say that ultimately compassionate leadership requires balance between showing empathy towards others but also knowing when to draw the line. West (2021, p. 5) states that 'compassionate leadership may be mistaken for a soft and an ineffective approach to leading', going on to say that more 'courage is required to lead compassionately than to lead using command and control'. 'Compassion can be reduced if a staff member fears they will be viewed as weak or vulnerable for giving or receiving compassion' (West 2021, p. 68). Pezaro et al.'s (2024) international, appreciative inquiry, entitled *Characteristics of strong midwifery leaders and enablers of strong midwifery leadership: An international appreciative inquiry*, challenges the assumption that compassionate leadership is weak leadership. The study used an online cross-sectional survey, with 429 participants from 76 countries. One of the findings that compassion is seen as an essential characteristic of the strong midwifery leader 'adds to an understanding of the importance of compassionate leadership' (Pezaro et al. 2024). Importantly, Pezaro et al. (2024) give a definition of compassionate leadership *in midwifery* as 'the combination of supportive leadership approaches, combined with West and Chowla's (2017) four pillars of compassion: attending, understanding, empathising, and helping'. The participants of the study reflected that compassionate leadership enabled psychologically safer working environments, positive cultures, midwives enjoying going to work, with leaders being seen as 'approach-able, kind and prioritising the well-being of staff' (Pezaro et al. 2024). It is impor-tant to note that Jacinda Arden, previous Prime Minister of New Zealand, strongly believes that as a leader, it is possible to be both compassionate and strong:

> One of the criticisms I've faced over the years is that I'm not aggressive enough or assertive enough or maybe somehow because I'm empathetic it means I'm weak. I totally rebel against that. I refuse to believe that you cannot be both compassionate and strong. (Dowd 2018)

Certainly, when implementing successful culture change, it is necessary for com-passionate leaders in maternity and neonatal services to be both strong and compas-sionate; to be compassionate in a negative culture requires much strength. The compassionate leadership theory, involving the four elements of attending, under-standing, empathising and helping, appears quite simple and straightforward, but implementing them is not; it requires ongoing intentional practice, attention and commitment (Ledger 2021). The King's Fund, in their document, *The courage of compassion: Supporting nurses and midwives to deliver high quality care*, calls upon health and care environments to 'have compassionate leadership and nurturing cultures that enable both care and staff support to be high-quality, continually improving and compassionate' (West et al. 2020), recognising that compassionate leadership requires courage.

> It requires the courage of compassionate leadership from all leaders, at every level of our health and care systems across the four UK countries, to engage with and successfully address the challenges that nursing and midwifery services face. Doing so is critical to our ability to care for the health and wellbeing of everyone across the United Kingdom. (West et al. 2020)

Both compassionate leadership and inclusion have been identified as 'golden threads of change' (OED 2025) (see Sects. 1.5 and 2.4), both essential to achieving positive maternity and neonatal cultures. To be inclusive, a leader must be compas-sionate. In a hospital, unit or department led by a compassionate leader, everyone will be included regardless of professional background, opinion, skin colour, sexu-ality, religion, gender, nationality, age, political views, disability, socioeconomic background, ethnicity or any other version of diversity, while taking account of neurodiverse preferences. Culture plays an important role in how compassion, as an emotional or cognitive process, is experienced and expressed; for example, the way in which a person behaves may be perceived differently by people of different cul-tures (Koopmann-Holm and Tsai 2017). As an example, Papadopoulos et al. (2021) cites Groark (2008) to explain some societies (e.g. Micronesian and Mayan) highly value secrecy and privacy, meaning that empathetic-like knowledge could be per-ceived as an intrusion or an attack.

> Culturally competent compassion in health care has been defined as a human quality of understanding the suffering of others and wanting to do something about it using culturally appropriate and acceptable caring interventions which take into consideration both the

patients' and the carers' cultural background as well as the context in which care is given. (Papadopoulos et al. 2021)

Leaders who display cultural sensitivity are aware of and respect cultural differences. They acknowledge that diverse cultures exist and understand the variations within them; they acquire specific knowledge and attitudes about another culture, which enables them to behave appropriately and effectively within that cultural context. However, cultural sensitivity can 'sometimes inadvertently imply an understanding of another's culture through our own lens and interpretations' (Barley 2022). To achieve cultural humility goes further by requiring us to 'approach others' cultures with humility, recognising our understanding will always be limited and evolving'. Self-awareness is the first step towards cultural humility, as it encourages leaders to examine their own cultural identities and biases or prejudices they may have (Barley 2022). Leaders who are compassionate and inclusive have a deep awareness of their cultural values, enabling them to understand how their own culture influences their leadership styles (Papadopoulos et al. 2021). To be culturally humble involves an ongoing process of learning and understanding, acknowledging personal biases and prejudices, and developing and maintaining respectful relationships to create an environment of respect (see Sect. 3.6).

Compassionate leadership creates psychological safety where staff feel safe to speak out about errors, problems and uncertainties (West 2021). When teams have compassionate leadership and, inevitably, psychological safety, maternity and neonatal staff are supported to vocalise thoughts, ideas and concerns without fear of retribution and blame (Edmondson 2018). This results in a culture of learning and innovation, with the organisation experiencing reduced levels of stress, errors, staff injuries, harassment, bullying and violence against staff, staff absenteeism and patient mortality (West 2021; West et al. 2014; Lyubovnikova et al. 2015).

> Compassionate leadership is ... at the heart of our efforts to nurture cultures that provide high-quality, continually improving and compassionate care for patients and service users. West 2021, p. 8).

The driver for writing this book began with working as a regional officer for the RCM, representing midwives who required support for employment and/or professional issues. It soon became clear that previously high-performing and motivated midwives who had or were being bullied, either by managers or colleagues quickly lost confidence, often went off sick and many were unable to go back into the workplace, with some never practising again. This was upsetting to observe, particularly as some midwives were subjected to disciplinary hearings because they had made poor decisions in psychologically unsafe environments. Very often, the reason midwives made mistakes was that they had lost confidence in their practice, became reluctant to make decisions and often were 'scared' to ask opinions of their colleagues. An anonymous true example of this is given in the vignette below:

**Box 7.2 Vignette: An Example of Poor Decision Making in the Absence of Compassionate Leadership and Psychological Safety**

Joanna (pseudonym), a midwife who had been qualified for three years, had spent most of that time as a 'rotating midwife', working between wards and departments to gain experience in all areas of midwifery. Joanna enjoyed midwifery and putting women and birthing people at the centre of care. She was keen to offer physiological third stage to women and birthing people, if this was their choice, following an informed discussion. This had become difficult to achieve because some senior midwives did not support physiological third stage and would stop Joanna discussing and implementing an informed choice policy when opportunities arose. As a result of this, Joanna began to lose confidence in her midwifery practice and had eventually stopped giving women and birthing people the option of a physiological third stage. There was one midwife, called Amanda, whom Joanna tried very hard not to work with because she was constantly criticising her practice, always in front of others. Joanna had begun to feel slightly anxious when driving to work when she was aware that Amanda was going to be on duty.

This particular day, Joanna drove to work for a late shift, in an anxious state, aware that Amanda was the birthing unit coordinator for that shift. Amanda allocated Joanna to care for a woman and birthing person called Rose; the midwife who had cared for Rose during the early shift needed to leave to attend a study afternoon. Joanna went into the room and immediately started to build a relationship with Rose and her partner. Initially all went well, it was Rose's first baby, and she was progressing well. Rose soon had an urge to 'push' and her cervix was confirmed to be fully dilated on vaginal examination. Rose was having strong contractions every four minutes and was pushing well. Joanna listened to the foetal heartbeat after every contraction and heard it to be within the normal range. After 30 minutes, the vertex was still not visible, and Joanna heard a deceleration of the baby's heartbeat after a contraction that recovered quickly. She went outside of the room to inform Amanda of this, who abruptly said she was extremely busy, this was a normal physiological process and to only inform her of serious problems. Joanna went back into the room and attached Rose to a cardiotocograph (CTG) monitor; the vertex was not visible, although Rose continued to push well; 20 minutes later, the foetal heart rate had begun to decelerate with and after each contraction, with the vertex still not visible. Joanna went to push the bell but suddenly, a wave of panic rushed over her at the thought of Amanda entering the room, she felt her heart rate accelerate and she felt sick. She knew that a different coordinator would be on duty in 30 minutes, *so she decided to wait until then.* As soon as the different coordinator arrived, Joanna rang the bell, but by this time, the baby was compromised, and Rose was urgently prepared for an emergency caesarean section. A baby girl was born in a poor condition, spending a week on the neonatal unit; a year later, all her milestones had been met, and she continues to be followed up by the paediatric service. A risk management

(continued)

> **Box 7.2** (continued)
>
> investigation was undertaken; the investigation took weeks and resulted in Joanna being referred to the Nursing and Midwifery Council (NMC) as the midwife who held accountability for Rose's care.
>
> Joanna received very little support from anyone on the unit during this time and eventually decided to resign before her case was heard at the NMC. She voluntarily removed herself from the midwives register because she was mentally unwell, culminating at one point in Rose considering taking her own life. Rose has not entered a maternity unit since the incident.

You may be asking why this vignette is placed in this section of the book. The answer is that it is an example of an incident that happened in a culture where compassionate leadership did not exist and staff did not feel psychologically safe. If this incident had occurred in a psychologically safe culture, led by compassionate leaders, Joanna would have felt safe to seek advice and care provided to Rose would have been safe.

When representing midwives, it soon became clear that some maternity units held very few disciplinary hearings and staff were complementary about their unit, whilst other units were often hearing disciplinary cases and grievances from unhappy staff. It became noticeable that one of the main differences between the units was leadership styles; units with few hearings and problems usually had leaders who displayed the elements of compassion, whilst the units experiencing problems often had autocratic, hierarchical leadership. The next section of this chapter explores the qualities of leaders who have successfully changed culture and actions they have taken that demonstrate compassionate leadership.

## 7.2.3  How Leaders Demonstrate Compassionate Leadership

Compassionate leadership is an essential 'golden thread' (OED 2025) in achieving positive culture change because it weaves through the 'golden threads' of respectful relationships, inclusion, values-based education, developing a coaching mindset, compassionate models of midwifery care, compassionate leadership and psychological safety. This section gives examples of compassionate leadership though the lens of successful leaders for whom the four elements of compassion, attending, understanding, empathising and helping (West and Bailey 2022; West 2021; West et al. 2017; West and Chowla 2017), are implicit within their leadership practice. The examples and opinions presented here are the views and experiences of compassionate leaders who are currently in or have held significant leadership roles across all four countries of the United Kingdom (UK). Some points were expressed by a majority and some by a minority, but all are examples of how they demonstrate compassionate leadership, particularly in relation to culture change. All leaders were passionate about midwifery and 'making it better' for women and birthing people and maternity and neonatal staff. Remember that in healthcare, everyone who champions, advocates and promotes care is a leader (Smith 2021; West 2021)) and, as such, has a responsibility for attending, understanding, empathising and helping others.

*Attending* means 'being present with, and attending to, those we lead. Leaders who attend will model being present with those they lead and listen 'with fascination'. Listening is one of the most important skills of leadership and involves taking the time to listen to the challenges, obstacles, frustrations and hurts of staff experience, as well as the successes and pressures'. (West 2021, p. 5). Listening is essential for compassionate leaders, enabling them to be present with and attend to staff they lead; to be able to speak honestly and openly, staff must feel 'safe' with their leaders as human beings and feel they are in a 'safe' environment in which to speak. This is particularly important for diverse staff members, as they 'need to feel safe to be themselves and be able to share the parts of their identity that they want to, but always by invitation not invasion' (Nadeem 2020). There are practical ways that compassionate leaders act to foster a feeling of psychological safety around them, thus creating an environment where staff feel safe and confident to be able to speak to them; leaders identified these actions as:

- Being clear and transparent.
- Staff must see you taking responsibility for and owning decisions.
- To be inclusive is essential, including using language that is inclusive and empowering.
- Demonstrating everyone is important, no matter who they are, including letting our students know we value them.
- Having an open-door policy, with staff knowing they can approach you to discuss issues at any time.
- If a staff member is asked to undertake a task and they make a mistake, it is important that you rectify the situation without blaming them.
- Having integrity.
- Accepting making mistakes should not be perceived as failure, and as a leader it is important to be open and honest about your mistakes and lessons learnt from them.
- Being courageous and having courageous conversations, *always challenge disrespectful behaviour** (every leader spoke about this).
- 'People need to believe in you'.
- If staff are going to share real issues, they must trust me.
- Everyone is given a voice and encouraged to speak up.
- You must be there in the room with your staff.
- Practice is very important in midwifery, and you must be perceived to be credible.
- Kindness to each other is essential.
- Being authentic.
- Important to take a 'no blame' approach.
- I work a day once a month in uniform so that I am seen as a human being.
- Sometimes you don't need to do anything, just listening, understanding and helping.

- It is important to appear friendly and greet people even when you are having a bad day.
- Always speaking positively about staff and women and birthing people.
- When listening to staff, be curious and interested in what they are saying (this point aligns with Kline 2002 who describes 'listening with fascination' as listening without interruptions and with curiosity).
- If a staff member has a concern, for example, they are feeling they are being treated disrespectfully, it is important that any actions are followed up (when staff feel 'nothing ever happens', they will stop voicing their concerns [Kirkup 2015, 2022]).

The importance of listening attentively has previously been discussed and identified as a coaching skill by Helen Rogers and Denise Linay (see Sect. 5.2). If all maternity and neonatal units develop a coaching mindset, as suggested by Helen and Denise, listening and empathy would be embedded into the culture, aligning with compassionate behaviour and leadership. A compassionate leader's role is to listen to understand someone's pain and take steps to alleviate it. However, a coach's role is not to rescue the coachee, but to support them in finding their own solution.

*Understanding* 'involves leaders appraising the situations those they lead are struggling with, to arrive at a measured understanding. Ideally leaders arrive at their understanding through dialogue with those they lead, which may involve reconciling conflicting perspectives rather than imposing their own understanding' (West 2021, p. 5).

Once staff have been genuinely listened to, it is essential that an agreed understanding is reached so that innovation, change and, ultimately, maternity and neonatal care are of the highest possible quality. Problems arise when there is a gap of understanding between the leaders of a service and the staff; the wider the gap, the bigger the problems become. The situation becomes more complex when there is also misunderstanding between the staff, who may perceive their problems differently. Sometimes, leaders believe that they have listened, but have not understood the situation; in these circumstances, staff believe that they have not been heard and consequently that leaders do not understand their problems (West 2021). Autocratic leaders would impose their own understanding of the situation and cause more disharmony, whereas compassionate leaders ensure that an agreed understanding of all parties is reached. As with 'attending', it is essential the environment is not only 'safe' for 'listening' but also safe for reconciling and difficult conversations to occur; the following is a list of actions compassionate leaders take to enable this.

- Respectful relationships are always maintained.
- Give people time to be courageous.
- You must not change your behaviour to make staff like you.
- Use examples of own experiences to make a point; one leader spoke about her own unconscious bias to emphasise its importance during training.
- Acknowledge the work everyone does.
- How you talk to people is important.

- All allegations of a member of staff being treated disrespectfully must be investigated.
- Understand peoples' differences and values.
- Have an open mind and be non-judgemental.
- You are not scared to make difficult decisions and will compromise when necessary.
- Work with the staff for as long as it takes to come to an understanding of the problem.
- Explain the reasons behind any difficulties that are being encountered.
- Focus on values and not on saving money.
- Sometimes, take a step back to give everyone an opportunity to participate.
- All ideas are considered.
- Encourage staff to challenge and value different opinions.
- Dignity is always maintained, especially during conflict.
- Always maintain confidentiality when staff discuss problems in their personal life with you.

*Empathising*: 'compassionate leadership requires being able to feel the distress or frustration of those we lead without being overwhelmed by the emotions and unable to help. Putting oneself in the other's shoes means taking their perspective which increases understanding of the sources and context of the difficulties they face' (West et al. 2011).

Feeley (2023, p. 45) describes empathy as 'the ability to understand the experiences and feelings of others outside of our own perspectives, it is an emotional skill that discerns between the emotions of ourselves and others and broadly is understanding, sharing and caring about the emotions of other people'. When a leader is empathetic towards those they lead, staff are more motived to find solutions to the challenges they face; 'feeling valued, respected, understood and supported by leaders fosters staff engagement and innovation' (West and Richer 2007). The following is a list of qualities and actions compassionate leaders described, demonstrating empathy to their staff:

- I try to be aware if I find myself treating someone less favourably and to be aware of any unconscious bias that I might have. For example, I suddenly realised that I had a negative opinion of anyone who had a lip piercing and realised I did think of them differently to everyone else.
- I am aware that people's unconscious bias has preconceived ideas of Black women, which includes women and staff.
- Find out what each midwife is good at and try to develop that skill.
- We developed a new model for practice; it was important that every midwife contributed.
- It is important to listen; sometimes people don't want answers, they just need to talk, and then they come up with the answers themselves.
- It is important to set boundaries, you can help someone more if you are not emotional, but that is something I find difficult.
- Leaders need to give people time to be courageous.

- Leaders who 'know' their staff are aware of their strengths and are able to inspire them.
- Leaders should allow themselves to be vulnerable.
- We arrange debriefs after all clinical incidents and arrange for midwives to meet with their professional midwifery advocate (PMA) if they want to.
- We organised a workshop, agreed what our acceptable and unacceptable behaviours were and every midwife signed up to them.
- I role-modelled a compassionate leader and now I am a leader myself, implementing the same ethos and values that I learnt from her.
- We have to be honest about when we are not OK; a lot of staff find that hard because they believe it would be seen as a failure.

*Helping*: 'probably the most important task of leaders in healthcare is to help those they lead to deliver the high-quality compassionate care they want to provide. Leadership, according to all definitions, includes helping and supporting others; helping means removing the obstacles that get in the way of people doing their work and providing the resources (staff, equipment and training for example) for them to do so' (Lilius et al. 2011).

After listening, understanding and empathising with the problems staff face, the final element is helping, and this entails providing resources that will alleviate suffering; it can mean anything from making somebody a cup of tea, to strongly advocating for extra staff in times of staff shortages. It can also mean leading a culture change to improve negative staff working environments, including challenging disrespectful behaviour and to encourage new and improved ways of working. Leaders gave examples of helping as:

- People who make other people scared to come to work must be dealt with through Human Resource (HR) processes.
- Staff must perceive you as kind, but equally, they must know that if someone crosses the line with the way in which they behave, for instance, you will take a hard line when necessary.
- Be radical and bold in finding solutions.
- Sometimes, improvements take for ever and staff 'give up' while waiting; our job is to change the processes to speed it all up.
- You lose credibility if you don't come up with the goods in the end.
- After COVID, all our staff were so tired, we arranged a 'wellness' week and organised different practitioners to come and give staff different treatments.
- We have organised a programme of coaching for midwives; it was hard to get the money for it, but it has really been worth it.
- All staff have received unconscious bias training.
- I am trying to get all staff to challenge poor behaviour; my motto is 'if you permit, you promote'.
- I identified my own learning and made sure I got it; you cannot help others if you do not help yourself.
- Schwartz Rounds have been implemented; they have made a big difference.

- You do need experience in writing bids, for example, for making the case for an increase in your staffing budget and be confident to present your case to the Trust Board,

---

**Box 7.3 Case-Study Example of Changing a Team's Culture Using Attributes of Compassionate Leadership**

Edna (pseudonym) was promoted into a new role within the same organisation and became the team leader of six professionals, who had been without a leader for six months; sharing the role between them on a monthly, rotational basis. The team had a reputation of being unapproachable, critical of each other and of other professionals, with two members of the team ostracised from the rest of the group, meaning they were often nervous to go to work, with high sickness rates. The professional team ran a community clinic, which received complaints from patients regarding staff being abrupt, their appointments sometimes delayed and cancelled. Edna soon realised that the team was dysfunctional and knew that it was crucial to change the working culture of the team; she made a decision to use the four elements of the theory of compassionate leadership (West et al. 2017).

*Attending*: To achieve the first element, Edna wanted the team members to feel safe to speak up, so decided to listen to their issues for the first few weeks by:

- Meeting with the six team members individually and listening with fascination (Kline 2002); it soon became clear that all the team members were unhappy with two very close to resigning and one team member 'off sick' on a regular basis.
- Having weekly meetings with the team, making it clear that everyone was to be treated with respect, everyone was equal and there was no hierarchy. During the meetings, everyone was given space and encouraged to speak and have an opinion.

Edna recognised the need to be supportive and was clear that she had an 'open-door policy' to give team members a chance to speak with her when they needed to.

*Understanding*: To achieve the second element, it was necessary for Edna to understand the issues and problems the team faced. Initially, there was a gap in her understanding of the way in which some of the team members behaved, so she realised that the understanding phase would take a while to achieve. Edna spent a day a week working with each team member to help her understand the pressures they faced. It soon became clear to her that everyone was working from a different page and there was a difference in

(continued)

Box 7.3 (continued)

understanding of each person's role within the team. There was no administrative support for the clinics, meaning that each clinic was chaotic, with each team member often working extra hours to complete paperwork.

*Empathy*: The third element of empathy was achieved because Edna took enough time to listen and gain an understanding of individual team members, enabling her to understand the issues the team faced. She was then able to have empathetic conversations with each team member, demonstrating an understanding of their situation but at the same time able to maintain her own position of everyone being treated respectfully was not negotiable. To achieve this position, Edna maintained eye contact, established a connection with the team member using verbal tone, body language and facial expression to establish a feeling of psychological safety.

*Helping*: The fourth and final element of compassionate leadership was achieved because Edna has listened, understood and empathised with the different team members, establishing their trust and belief that improvements could be made. Edna undertook a review of the roles and responsibilities of each team member, achieving a joint understanding of what was expected. She discussed the most appropriate education and training for each team member and organised coaching for them all. She acknowledged, with no blame, that team members did not always respect each other. Values for the team were agreed with everyone expected to uphold them; it was also agreed that disrespectful behaviour would be challenged as it occurred. Finally, Edna presented a business case to the Trust Board, achieving funding for an administrator for the clinic. Within nine months of being in post, Edna was pleased that the team were enjoying work and respecting each other, had received coaching, customer service training, a new administrator had commenced work and, most importantly, the complaints received from patients had reduced by two-thirds.

The case study below is a true account of how a leader changed a culture within a dysfunctional group of professional staff, using the four elements of West et al.'s (2017) theory of compassionate leadership: attending, listening, empathy and helping.

## 7.3 Conclusion

At the beginning of this chapter, we challenged you to reflect on your own leadership style and asked what you believed compassionate leadership is. We then described West's (2021) compassionate leadership theory consisting of four elements of attending, listening, empathising and helping, and challenged the misconception that compassionate leadership is weak leadership. We established that compassionate and inclusive leaderships are synonymous (West 2021) and if psychological safety is present, staff will feel safe to speak out about errors, problems and uncertainties, creating safer clinical environments for maternity and neonatal staff and for women and birthing people and neonates.

Finally, please complete the exercise below asking if your understanding of compassionate leadership has changed and ask if you believe you are a compassionate leader.

> **Box 7.4 Exercise: Has Your Understanding of Compassionate Leadership Changed?**
>
> Please answer the following questions:
>
> What do you think compassionate leadership is?
> Has this changed since reading this chapter?
> What do you think compassionate leadership looks like in midwifery practice? Has this changed since reading this chapter?
> Do you think you are a compassionate leader? If so, how do you attend, understand, empathise and help?

# References


Barley A (2022) Yorkshire Consortium for Equity in Doctoral Education. Cultural humility: A core skill for Inclusive Leadership in UK Higher Education. Available: https://ycede.ac.uk/cultural-humility-a-core-skill-for-inclusive-leadership-in-uk-higher-education/#:~:text=Cultural%20Humility%20as%20a%20Core,on%20research%20inquiries%20and%20methodologies. (accessed 24 Feb 2025)

Brown B (2025) The power of vulnerability in leadership Education Support. Available: https://www.educationsupport.org.uk/resources/for-organisations/articles/the-power-of-vulnerability-in-leadership/ (Accessed 25 Feb 2025)

Dowd M (2018) Lady of the Rings: Jacinda Arden. New York Times. Available: https://www.nytimes.com/2018/09/08/opinion/sunday/jacinda-ardern-new-zealand-prime-minister.html (Accessed 25 Feb 2025)

Edmondson AC (2018) The Fearless Organization: Creating Psychological Safety in the Workplace for Learning, Innovation, and Growth. Wiley: New Jersey.

Feeley C (2023) Skilled Heartfelt midwifery Practice. Safe, Relational Care for Alternative Physiological Births. Springer, Switzerland Available https://doi.org/10.1007/978-3-031-43643-7 (accessed 7 Feb 2025)

Groark K P (2008) Social opacity and the dynamics of empathic in-sight among the Tzotzil Maya of Chiapas, Mexico. Ethos, 36(4), 427–448. https://doi.org/10.1111/j.1548-1352.2008.00025.x

Kaufman (2023) The Power of compassionate Leadership Available: https://kariekaufmann.com/compassionate-leadership/ (Accessed 4 Feb 2025)

Kirkup B (2022) Reading the signals, Maternity and Neonatal Services East Kent – the report of the independent investigation. London: His Majesty's Stationary Office. Available: https://assets.publishing.service.gov.uk/media/634fb083e90e0731a5423408/reading-the-signals-maternity-and-neonatal-services-in-east-kent_the-report-of-the-independent-investigation_print-ready.pdf (accessed 28 Jan 2025)

Kirkup B (2015) The Report of the Morecambe Bay Investigation. Available: http://data.parliament.uk/DepositedPapers/Files/DEP2015-0267/The_Report_of_the_Morecambe_Bay.pdf (Accessed 27 January 2025)

Kline N (2002) Time to Think, Listening to Ignite the Human Mind. Ward Lock, Cassell Illustrated, London

Koopmann-Holm, B., & Tsai, J. L. (2017). The cultural shaping of compassion. In E. M. Seppälä, E. Simon-Thomas, S. L. Brown, M. C. Worline, C. D. Cameron, & J. R. Doty (Eds.), Oxford handbook of compassion science (pp. 273–285). Oxford University Press

Ledger K (2021) Person–Centered and Compassionate Leadership, In J Smith (Ed) Nurturing Maternity Staff. How to tackle trauma, stress and burnout to create a positive working culture in the NHS. (pp. 44–60) Pinter and Martin, UK

Lilius JM, Kanov J, Dutton JE, Worline MC, Maitlis S (2011) Compassion revealed: what we know about compassion at work (and where we need to know more). In Cameron KS, Spreitzer GM (Eds). The Oxford handbook of positive organisational scholarship pp 273–287 Oxford University Press, New York

Lyubovnikova J, West M A, Dawson J F, and Carter M R (2015) 24-Karat or fool's gold? Consequences of real team and co-acting group membership in healthcare organizations. European Journal of Work and Organizational Psychology, 24(6), 929–950. https://doi.org/10.1080/1359432X.2014.992421

Nadeem S (2020) Being an inclusion ally. Care Quality Commission, London

NHS England (2025) NHS Leadership Academy. Available: https://www.leadershipacademy.nhs.uk/ accessed 26 Feb 2025

Oxford English Dictionary (2025) Oxford University Press. Oxford Available at: https://www.oxfordlearnersdictionaries.com/definition/english/golden-thread?q=golden+thread (Accessed 28 Feb 2025)

Pezaro S, Zarbiv G, Jones J, Lilei Feika M, Fitzgerald L, Lukhele S, Mcmillan-Bohler J, Baloyi OB, Maravic da Silva K, Grant C, Bayliss-Pratt L, Hardtman P (2024) Characteristics of strong midwifery leaders and enablers of strong midwifery leadership: An international appreciative inquiry. Midwifery. https://doi.org/10.1016/j.midw.2024.103982 Available: https://www.sciencedirect.com/science/article/pii/S0266613824000664?via%3Dihub (Accessed 24 Feb 2025)

Papadopoulos I, Lazzarino R, Koulouglioti C, Aagard M, Akman O, Alpers L-M, Apostolara P, Araneda-Berna J, Biglete-Pangilina S, Eldar-Regev O, et al (2021). The Importance of being a compassionate leader: the views of nursing and midwifery managers from around the world. 32(6), 765–777. Available: https://journals.sagepub.com/doi/full/10.1177/10436596211008214 (Accessed 26 Feb 2025)

RCM (2021) The Solution Series: 2 Making Maternity Services Safer: The Role of Leadership Available: https://uat.rcm.org.uk/media/5064/the-solution-series-2-making-maternity-services-safer-the-role-of-leadershippdf (Accessed 24 Feb 2025) thae-solution-series-2-making-maternity-services-safer-the-role-of-leadershippdf h

Smith J (2021) Nurturing Maternity Staff. How to tackle trauma, stress and burnout to create a positive working culture in the NHS. Pinter and Martin, UK

The Kings Fund (2025) Ideas that change health and care. Available: https://www.kingsfund.org.uk/ (Accessed 24 Feb 2025)

West MA, Bailey S (2022) What is Compassionate Leadership The Kings Fund https://www.kingsfund.org.uk/insight-and-analysis/long-reads/what-is-compassionateleadership (Accessed 25 Feb 2025)

West MA (2021) Compassionate Leadership: Sustaining Wisdom, Humanity and Presence Health and Social Care. London: Swirling Leaf Press.

West MA, Bailey S, Williams E (2020) The courage of compassion Supporting nurses and midwives to provide high quality care. The Kings Fund. Available: https://www.kingsfund.org.uk/insight-and-analysis/reports/courage-compassion-supporting-nurses-midwives (Accessed 4 Feb 2025).

West M, Eckert R, Collins B, Chowla R, (2017) Caring to change: how compassionate leadership can stimulate innovation in health care 2017. The Kings Fund Available: https://assets.kingsfund.org.uk/f/256914/x/0b76247d02/caring_to_change_2017.pdf (Accessed 24 Feb 2025)

West MA and Chowla R (2017) Compassionate leadership for compassionate health care. in P Gilbert (ed.), Compassion: Concepts, Research and Applications. Routledge, London, pp. 237–257. Available: https://doi.org/10.4324/9781315564296 Accessed 26 Feb 2025

West MA, Lyubovnikova J, Eckert R, Denis J (2014) Collective leadership for cultures of high-quality healthcare. Journal of organisational effectiveness: People and Performance. 1(3), 240–250

West MA, Dawson JF, Admasachew L, Topakus A (2011) NHS staff management and health service quality; results from the NHS staff survey and related data. Report to the Department of Health and Social Care. Available: https://assets.publishing.service.gov.uk/media/5a7c8b0eed915d6969f459d5/dh_129656.pdf Accessed 24 Feb 2025

West MA, Richer AW (2007) Climates and coaches for innovation and creativity at work. In Ford C, (ed) Handbook of organisational creativity pp 211–237; Taylor and Francis, London

Worline MC, Boik S (2006) Leadership lessons from Sarah: values based leadership as everyday practise. In Cameron K, Hess E (Eds) Leading with values: Positivity, virtue and high performance pp 108–131 Cambridge University press, Cambridge

# Finding Resolution

**8**

Maggie O'Brien

## 8.1 Introduction

This chapter draws together the 'golden threads of change' (OED 2025), identified within the book as essential to achieving positive maternity cultures in our workplaces (see Sect. 1.5). All 'golden threads of change' are interlinked, for example, to achieve respectful relationships; psychological safety must be in place for staff to feel able to raise concerns regarding disrespectful behaviour. When one element of a disrespectful culture improves, it will start to impact positively upon other elements. This chapter gives guidance on ways to achieve respectful relationships, inclusion, values-based education developing a coaching mindset, models of care, compassionate leadership and psychological safety as a means of achieving positive cultures, giving examples of how compassionate leaders have achieved culture change in the workplaces they are responsible for.

By completing the exercises throughout the book, you will have started to develop an understanding of whether you work in a compassionate workplace, have a compassionate leader and reflected on your own leadership style. To speak up and challenge disrespectful and possible bullying behaviour either towards yourself, or a colleague, within the hospital, maternity unit or department you work in, may seem overwhelming. You will not be alone, wherever you are placed in an organisation; to make any change requires courage and a passion to improve the well-being of yourself, colleagues you work with and quality of care and experience for women and birthing people. *The challenge to us all is to make a start, no matter how small that start may be.* Whether you are a senior manager, a member of maternity or neonatal staff, or a student, your start may be to decide to consciously be kind to yourself and/or in your everyday interactions with people; it may be to challenge

M. O'Brien (✉)
University of Southampton, Southampton, United Kingdom

Royal College of Midwives RCMF (Hons), London, United Kingdom
e-mail: Mahues935@gmail.com



M. O'Brien, E. Kitson-Reynolds (eds.), *Respectful Relationships in the Maternity Service*, https://doi.org/10.1007/978-3-032-04281-1_8

disrespectful behaviour, either directed at yourself or others, or it may be to lead a culture change programme. If change is required in your workplace, this chapter will encourage you to make that start and to help others to do so, no matter how big or small that change may be. We are aware that the quality of maternity care is variable (Care Quality Commission [CQC] 2024) (see Sect. 2.3), with some maternity units providing high-quality, compassionate care where culture change is not necessary; in these maternity units, it is important that staff continue to challenge disrespectful behaviour, making it unacceptable. People who work in positive cultures have 'bad days'; the advice in this chapter also applies to addressing disrespectful behaviour that is not part of a wider cultural problem.

## 8.2 Personal Strategies for Addressing Disrespectful Behaviour

This section provides guidance on how we can develop personal strategies to address disrespectful behaviour directed towards ourselves and/or others. The first step in being able to challenge disrespectful behaviour is the belief that the problem lies with the perpetrator and has nothing to do with anything you may or may not have done (O'Brien 2018b). People who treat others with disrespect often target innovative, compassionate individuals who are passionate about creating positive cultures. The tall poppy syndrome discussed previously (see Sect. 2.7) explains how inspirational, innovative, motivated people are often the first to be targeted or chopped down, just as tall poppies are the first to be harvested in the field. The problem is, even tall poppies cannot stand the pressure of constant criticism, being ostracised and humiliated so either are forced to change their behaviour or decide to leave (Elliott 2004). The following quote describes the process that occurs:

> Workplace abusers lie, misusing their power to silence your truth so they can weaken you, push you out, and no longer feel threatened by your competence. (End Workplace Abuse 2025)

If you are being subject to disrespectful behaviour, try to find the courage and strength to challenge it, using the strategies described below to help you.

**Identifying Whether You Are Being Bullied** Identify whether the behaviour directed at you is bullying, harassment, discrimination or victimisation (see Sect. 2.7). Gillen et al.'s (2004) concept analysis identified the four defining attributes of bullying behaviour that must be present if bullying has occurred; as a reminder, these are as follows:

1. The repeated nature of the behaviour.
2. Negative effect of the behaviour on the victim.
3. The victim finds it difficult to defend themselves (power imbalance).
4. Intent of the bully.

**Make It Clear to Anyone Who Displays Disrespectful and/or Bullying Behaviour Towards You That You Will Not Accept It** It is much easier to write than to implement but is extremely important and may be the first step towards transforming yours and others' working lives. Because bullying relies on a power imbalance (Gillen et al. 2004) and 'fear is often the driver behind exerting power over people' (Smith 2021, p. 107), it is important to demonstrate that you are not afraid of the person treating you with disrespect; by making this clear, you will address the power imbalance. To achieve this, the first time you are treated with disrespect, say something like 'why did you speak to me like that?' or 'please do not speak to me like that again'. Once you have summoned the courage to challenge the behaviour, it is unlikely (not certain) that person will treat you with disrespect again (O'Brien 2018b, c). Disrespectful behaviour should be challenged as soon as possible after it occurs, because once a power imbalance is established, it is more difficult to challenge unacceptable behaviour.

**What Happens if I Cannot Challenge the Behaviour** If you are unable to challenge the behaviour, or you are aware that the person targets and treats others with disrespect, it is important that you report it, so that it can be formally addressed. What you decide to do will often depend on how psychologically safe you feel; within positive, safe environments, it will be accepted practice to challenge and report unacceptable behaviour, but sadly, fear of speaking up (Kirkup 2015, 2022; RCM 2016), of becoming the next victim and a fear that nothing will be done (Aunger et al. 2023) means that reporting bullying does not always occur (see Sect. 3.4.1). The Royal College of Midwives (RCM) Survey of the Health, Safety and Wellbeing of Midwives and Maternity Support Workers found that 37% of midwives who had experienced bullying did not report it (RCM 2017). This fact is as concerning as the bullying itself, because failure to report bullying usually means that staff do not feel psychologically safe. It is recommended you contact your trade union/professional organisation representative to obtain advice and support before reporting the behaviour. Keep a record of all the incidents where you are treated disrespectfully, including the dates and times and make a note of any witnesses to the behaviour. In the first instance, you should report the behaviour to the person's manager, your Head of Midwifery (HOM) or contact Human Resources (HR) and discuss with them; most National Health Service (NHS) Trusts and private healthcare organisations have Bullying and Harassment policies designed to address bullying and it is possible to lodge a grievance, as a final resort, as discussed below. If there is no one within your maternity or neonatal unit you feel comfortable to report the unacceptable behaviour to, consider speaking to your Trust's Freedom to Speak Up Guardian. NHS England's 'Freedom to Speak Up Policy for the NHS' (NHS England 2022) gives details of whom you can speak to within your NHS Trust and is a policy accessible to all staff and students.

**Support Anyone You Believe Is Being Treated Disrespectfully and/or Bullied** A person who is being targeted will often believe that they are to blame; therefore, if you witness bullying behaviour towards them by speaking up, you can give them confidence to challenge the person. If circumstances make this impossible, taking the person aside and privately saying you witnessed the behaviour can often make a difference in restoring their self-esteem, well-being and give them confidence to challenge the behaviour by speaking up for themselves (O'Brien 2018b, c).

> Reaching in to our colleagues, and those we support is not about absorbing their difficulties, stresses, or problems—rather, it's about connecting with them to say: 'I see you, I am here for you, and you matter'. The smallest of actions we show to others can be embedded into their psyche as 'I am valued'. (Smith 2021, p. 27)

When a culture of compassion and support is established, and staff feel psychologically safe, it becomes difficult and unacceptable to treat someone with disrespect.

**Obtain Support and Advice from Trade Unions/Professional Bodies**  If you are not a member of a trade union/professional body, it is recommended that you join one; this could be the RCM (RCM 2025), the Royal College of Nursing (RCN), (RCN 2025), UNISON (UNISON 2025) or your own trade union/professional body. The RCM and RCN are both professional bodies and trade unions (O'Brien 2022, p. 23), with the RCM being the first professional organisation to affiliate with the Trade Union Congress (TUC), an organisation who lobby actively for equality and employment rights (TUC 2025). UNISON is a trade union that represents public service workers. The trade union/professional body that you choose to join will provide representation for future employment issues, but will not be able to represent you for past issues that occurred when you were not a member.

**Be Aware of Your Organisation's Grievance Policy**  Unless you work in a self-employed capacity, every organisation providing healthcare in the United Kingdom (UK) should have a grievance policy that can be initiated if you believe that you are being bullied or harassed. You can discuss how lodging a grievance would apply to your situation with HR and/or your trade union representative. The grievance policy will provide a framework, guidance and time frame for the process, which usually involves an investigation, followed by a hearing, where both parties have the opportunity to present their 'case'. Your trade union representative will represent and support you through the process; they will also provide advice if you believe that you are being harassed or victimised (RCM 2025; RCN 2025; UNISON 2025). The grievance procedure can be a stressful process for everyone involved and it is recommended that lodging a grievance should be considered as a final resort. However, by lodging a grievance, attention is brought to the wider organisation of a situation that may be being ignored within the maternity or neonatal unit senior management team.

**Seek Help and Support from Someone That You Trust and/or Professional Midwifery Advocate (PMA)**  If you believe you are being targeted, it is important you speak to a trusted friend, colleague or a member of your family (O'Brien

2018b). To ignore it and *just carry on* can have a significant impact on your mental and physical health (see Sect. 2.7.5); the person you choose to talk to will be able to support you to challenge this behaviour and help you understand you are not to blame and did nothing to deserve it. If you are a midwife or a student midwife, a person to be considered to discuss your situation with is a PMA (Kitson-Reynolds 2020; Kerelo 2020); these are a team or group of midwives appointed by your local NHS maternity service to support midwives through their professional development by using the A-equip model (NHS England 2017).

**Support for Students**  If you are a student who believes you are being treated disrespectfully or bullied, you can access support and advice through your university or the NHS Trust where you are undertaking your clinical placements. There is international and UK evidence (see Sect. 2.2) that some student midwives are bullied, usually by a midwife, whilst on clinical placement and less frequently by university lecturers and personal tutors (Gillan et al. 2008; Gillen et al. 2009; Catling et al. 2017; Capper 2021; Wylam 2023; McNeil and Kitson-Reynolds 2024). There have been a few occasions where students feel that they are being treated badly by other members of their cohort. If you belong to the RCM, RCN, the Student Union or another trade union, they should be your first port of call for support, advice and representation if required; this applies whether the advice you require relates to the university or NHS Trust. If you are being treated disrespectfully whilst on clinical placement, discuss this with your practice assessor or supervisor, the manager of the area in which the person works or the HOM. Within your university, it is recommended that you approach your personal tutor for support and advice; they may suggest that you approach the manager of the person involved together. It can often help to discuss the issue with trusted members of your cohort who will be able to support you, and you may find that other students have had or are having similar issues. You will have access to a PMA, with all PMAs available to support students in practice (Kitson-Reynolds 2022; Kerelo 2020); your local PMA team may comprise practising midwives across the clinical service and the university teaching team (see Sect. 4.3). You also have access to the NHS Trust's Freedom to Speak Up Guardian (NHS England 2022). If you are being treated disrespectfully by a member of the university teaching team, your personal tutor or by another student or students within your cohort, speak to someone whom you trust within the university. If you are not comfortable to speak to your personal tutor, you can speak to your programme lead for midwifery education, academic assessor, another member of the teaching team, or, if available, a PMA within your university. Support for students will be provided by your university, usually through a confidential hub, that can be accessed independently, that you are able to approach for confidential advice and, in most cases, counselling. As with NHS Trusts, universities have policies to address bullying and harassment behaviour and it is possible to lodge a grievance; if you decided to do this, it is recommended that you obtain the support of a trade union representative.

**Above All Else, Demonstrate Self-Compassion and Be Kind to Yourself** If you are being treated with disrespect, it is particularly important that you practise self-compassion to help protect your mental and physical health. The Nursing and Midwifery Council (NMC) recognises and reinforces the importance of self-compassion for midwives within Domain 5 in the Standards for 'Pre-registration Midwifery Programmes', by stating '...midwives should incorporate compassionate self-care into their personal and professional life' (NMC 2019). The following is a definition of self-compassion given by Michael West the ethos of which, perhaps we should all aspire to achieve for ourselves:

> Self-compassion means being warm, self-soothing and understanding towards ourselves in situations where we suffer, behave badly or 'fail' rather than denying our pain or beating ourselves up Self-compassion involves a recognition that being imperfect, failing and experiencing life difficulties is inevitable. (West 2021, p. 208)

It is recommended that you read the book *Nurturing Maternity Staff* (Smith 2021), particularly the chapter, *The Tide of Change* (Smith 2021, pp. 84–105) that gives excellent advice to staff and students on caring for themselves. People often think that self-care means going on holiday, retreats, having massages, etc., whereas it is often regenerating to do these things; self-care is much simpler than this. It is being kind to yourself, for example, saying 'no' to something you know will cause you stress and spending time with family and people who value you. Smith (2021, p. 101) suggests that many people find it hard to be kind to themselves, recommending we start in small, simple ways such as ensuring that we have a drink of water when we are thirsty or a snack when hungry. Smith (2021) also recommends that when your mind is loud and being unkind, try and generate self-compassion, as described by Michael West above. If you have been physically and/or mental affected by workplace bullying (see Sect. 2.7.5), do not ignore it; it is important that you consult your General Practitioner (GP) and obtain treatment and/or help if necessary. To acknowledge you need support and help, sometimes because of circumstances outside of your control, and then to seek help, requires great courage (Smith 2021, p. 87). If you find yourself working in a culture that is counter to your own values and/or your behaviour and the way in which you practise is changing, perhaps causing an adverse effect on your mental health, sometimes, the only way to be self-compassionate is to resign from that particular NHS Trust or organisation. All maternity and neonatal services have different cultures; if you are able to move, you will probably find a maternity or neonatal service that aligns with your own values. As hard as it may be, it is important to make this decision because your confidence, self-esteem, mental and/or physical health may be impacted in the long term (Fig. 8.1).

If you are unsure of what to do, need advice, support and/or representation contact your trade union/professional body

Determine if the behaviour is disrespectful, bullying, harassment or victimisation

Keep a record of all incidents that occur, including dates and times and any witnesses

Challenge the behaviour, if possible, when, or as soon as possible after it occurs

If possible, report the behaviour to the person's manager, your HOM or discuss with HR

Support anyone you know is being treated disrespectfully

Speak to someone you trust for *support*, this could be a PMA, work colleague, family member, personal friend and be aware of possible physical/mental health symptoms, gaining help through your GP, if necessary

Students in the UK may approach the following for support and/or advice:
    RCM/RCN/Student Union/UNISON representatives.
    University personal tutor, academic assessor, lecturers, Head of Programme.
    University student wellbeing centre/hub.
    NHS Trust assessor, supervisor, manager of area, HOM.
    NHS Trust/University PMA
    NHS Trust Freedom to Speak Up Guardian.

Practice self-compassion and be kind to yourself.

**Fig. 8.1** Summary of actions to address disrespectful behaviour towards yourself

## 8.3    Advice and Examples Given by Compassionate Leaders to Achieve Positive Maternity and Neonatal Cultures

This section uses the 'golden threads of change' (OED 2025) as a framework to summarise experiences and advice given by inspirational, compassionate leaders on how they have achieved the implementation and maintenance of positive workplace cultures.

### 8.3.1    Achieving Respectful Relationships

**Make Disrespectful and Bullying Behaviour Unacceptable**  This point was made by every leader spoken to, all of whom believe that a zero tolerance towards bullying behaviour is essential to achieving respectful relationships. To enforce a zero-tolerance philosophy requires courage, determination and credibility plus a commitment to taking all allegations of bullying seriously by the entire management team (O'Brien 2018b). To report incidents of bullying, staff must have a belief that they will be taken seriously, and confidentiality will be respected; this is because the fear experienced by the 'victim' and 'bystanders' cannot be underestimated. Remember that cultures develop around staff members who abuse power (see Sect. 2.7), with other staff changing their behaviour to 'fit in' (Baumeister and Leary 1995; Hadikin and O'Driscoll 2000; Hunter 2005). The longer the culture has been in place, the more toxic it will become. When their power base is threatened, staff at the centre of the culture will try to exert more power to maintain their position

(O'Brien 2018b). Therefore, if cultures are to change, a *zero-tolerance approach must be implemented and upheld, not only by leaders and managers but by all staff working within the area.* If it is known that some staff and students are scared to work with an individual, changing their shifts and going 'off sick' to avoid doing so, it is everyone's responsibility to acknowledge and report it in a professional manner to the individual's manager or HR.

> One of the key factors which would affect a change in the workplace be the expressed disapproval of colleagues. Bullying should be openly discussed at every opportunity, staff forums, in the canteen, during work and everyone should feel free to openly express their disapproval for such behaviour. (Hadikin and O'Driscoll 2000, p. 122)

From experience, bullies often have a free reign because of a reluctance of staff within the area to openly discuss it; this can be because bullies often use emotional manipulation to maintain their control and power, for example, being extremely 'nice' to someone one day and then openly criticising, ostracising and making hurtful comments, the next. The effect of this on the victim is to experience an emotional roller-coaster consisting of a cycle of fear, then relief, depending on the perpetrator's mood that day. Excuses should not be made for a person's unacceptable behaviour, for example, by saying, 'she always behaves like that, but is harmless, take no notice' (O'Brien 2018b, c); this person may be causing irreparable damage to someone's mental health, including affecting their ability to work in the long term. One leader described how she believed she managed all staff compassionately, but it was essential everyone believed that she would act immediately when 'someone crossed the line' and that staff knew if they behaved disrespectfully, there would be consequences.

**Co-create a Set of Acceptable and Non-acceptable Behaviours with Staff and Ensure That Everyone Adheres to Them** Several leaders discussed the importance of this, describing how it was achieved, emphasising the importance of involving *all staff in the process,* together with maternity and neonatal service user representatives. Once accepted and unaccepted behaviours are agreed with all staff, it becomes much easier to challenge unacceptable behaviour and so achieve respectful relationships.

---

**Box 8.1 Vignette: An Example of Achieving Respectful Relationships Through the Co-creation of a Behaviours Charter**

Judith is a HOM of a large maternity and neonatal service, situated within a city with 5 sites providing maternity and neonatal care, ranging from tertiary care to midwifery-led birthing units. Judith had become concerned about a growing number of concerns raised by some students and newly appointed midwives about a range of uncivil behaviours displayed in some areas, increasing sickness and absence related to stress and high attrition rates. In addition, the senior midwifery and neonatal management teams wanted to

(continued)

**Box 8.1** (continued)

positively respond to concerns and reports of poor morale, with the intention of building a culture of safety following the publication of the Independent Maternity Review (2022). The COVID-19 pandemic had caused increasing stress to all staff, there had been some acute staffing pressures and an increasing acuity and intervention rates over time had caused higher workloads and bed occupancy. Judith acknowledged that when staff work under stressful situations, there can be an impact on behaviour, but did not want uncivil behaviours to become normalised over time; so she decided the staff would spend time together, as a team, to pause and remind themselves of what they did and agree how they wanted to work together as a team.

To achieve this, the management team drew up a long list of potential enabling and constraining behaviours which were tested during a series of six sessions attended by about 70 staff, other ideas were added, cards were produced for all areas and placed in staff rooms. An online survey ran for a month, and overall, 200 staff responded, providing their views on acceptable and unacceptable behaviours. A Behaviours Charter was co-created, stating that staff would carry out the top ten positive/enabling behaviours as consistently as possible and not display or tolerate the top ten negative behaviours. The charters were displayed in all areas and an action plan was developed to decide how to make the charter part of everyday practice. Everyone became aware of the focus on behaviour, resulting in a reduction of reporting uncivil behaviour occurring quite quickly, with a slower but consistent reduction in sickness and absence rates.

**A Guide to Managing Disrespectful and Bullying Behaviour**  Anyone who has held a leadership and/or managerial position will be aware of how difficult this can be. To achieve positive culture change and for staff to believe in your determination to achieve a psychologically safe workplace, they must see a consistent commitment to addressing unacceptable behaviour and establishing zero intolerance of bullying. It is important that the whole leadership team take every allegation of disrespectful behaviour seriously, treating everyone compassionately and in the same way, following HR policies that exist within each organisation. When a member of staff makes an allegation of bullying, they must be taken seriously and treated with compassion; to achieve this, meet with the staff member and

*Attend* by listening deeply and quietly, so the person can explain themselves clearly and feel understood. Allow space for silence and reflection, as often the person will add more in the spaces (West 2021, p. 21). Listen to the details of the incidents of and of how they made the person feel.

*Understand* through 'listening with curiosity' to gain an understanding of the situation, for example, through determining if the type of behaviour displayed was disrespectful, bullying, harassment, victimisation or discrimination and finding out what actually happened through the lens of the victim.

*Empathy*: Demonstrate your empathy by understanding that the victim may be suffering mentally or physically and that providing psychological safety will be necessary; this may mean moving the perpetrator to another area until the process is complete.

*Helping* by bringing the process to completion as soon as possible and by arranging ongoing emotional support for the victim.

When meeting with the alleged perpetrator, address the behaviour not the person, 'our focus should be on not accepting the behaviours rather than not accepting the individual' (West 2021, p. 18) and as with the victim, treat the person with compassion. If the workplace has a set of agreed acceptable and unacceptable behaviours, as described above, there will be a sound basis on which to base your conversation. Remember that when faced with a culture of fear and intimidation, some midwives change their behaviour in order to 'fit-in' (see Sect. 2.7); when these midwives' behaviour is challenged, they usually express regret and immediately express concern for the person who has been impacted by their behaviour. In these circumstances, a meeting including the relevant manager, perpetrator and victim (supported by a trade union representative or colleague) usually resolves the issue and a way forward to treat everyone respectfully can be agreed by everyone.

However, if the allegation is against a staff member who holds the power, at the centre of the culture (see Sect. 2.7), the situation is more complex and will require much courage and compassionate leadership to resolve.

> Compassionate leadership creates the conditions where the needs of patients and staff, well-being and development are prioritised over individual agendas, aggression or undermining. (West 2021, p. 21)

Once the allegation has been made, it is essential to maintain psychological safety for all staff, as the person may make counter allegations of bullying and try to manipulate staff to provide evidence on their behalf, against the victim. For these reasons, the person may need to be moved to another area or suspended, whilst an investigation takes place. If suspension or a move is considered necessary, follow the organisation's correct procedure, together with obtaining the advice of HR. The alleged perpetrator should be advised to seek the support, advice and representation of their trade union/professional body. During the conversation, take the following compassionate approach:

*Attend* by listening deeply and quietly so the person can explain themselves clearly and feel understood. Allow space for silence and reflection, as often the person will add more in the spaces (West 2021, p. 21). As with the victim, it is essential to listen to gain an understanding of the situation through the lens of the perpetrator.

*Understand* by demonstrating you understand the situation from their perspective, including factors that may have been present when the alleged incidents of unacceptable behaviour occurred, for example, low staffing, high acuity, or personal issues such as bereavement.

*Empathy* through demonstrating an understanding of work and/or personal pressures that may have been present, but at the same time maintaining your own position that disrespectful and bullying behaviour is not acceptable and there is an expectation of staff to behave respectfully.

*Helping* by completing the process as soon as possible to reduce stress and by ensuring support for both individuals is available.

If anyone displays seriously abusive behaviour such as racism, sexual harassment or homophobia, you should consult HR and invoke the organisation's relevant policy, which will include the process to follow if a decision is made to suspend the person. The perpetrators of this behaviour must be treated fairly, with transparency and with clear time frames, but it is essential that abusive behaviour is not tolerated (West 2021).

---

**Box 8.2 Case Study: An Example of Addressing Disrespectful Behaviour to Achieve Respectful Relationships**

A new HOM was appointed to a maternity unit where she very quickly became aware that the staff worked in an environment of fear and intimidation, creating a culture where it was 'normal' to treat each other with disrespect. This resulted in high sickness levels and a very high staff turnover rate of 33% of junior grade midwives, plus a difficulty in recruiting new midwives, all of which contributed towards a high vacancy rate. There were a high number of complaints from women, which involved investigations into practice and behaviour and meetings with women and their families to reach resolution.

This culture had developed over many years, mainly because the senior midwives on the Birthing Unit had established a position of power, resulting in many midwives being frightened to work there, consequently, losing their midwifery skills and confidence. The situation became so serious that a grievance was submitted by a trade union on behalf of one of its members. The HOM, in consultation with human resources and the trade union, undertook a confidential investigation into the allegations of bullying and harassment. The investigation involved an independent manager interviewing 80 midwives and maternity care assistants who had worked on the Birthing Unit over the preceding two years. The most important factor was that the investigation was completely confidential; unless this was believed by the staff who were interviewed, they would not have spoken up, due to fear. The staff were asked the same questions and no 'leading questions' were asked. It was decided to ask all staff the following three questions:

(continued)

**Box 8.2** (continued)

1.  What do you enjoy about coming to work?
2.  What do you find less enjoyable about coming to work?
3.  What, if anything, would you change?

The findings of the investigation were that all the staff interviewed had been subjected to disrespectful and bullying behaviour and most had experienced the physiological, psychological and/or behavioural symptoms associated with this. The investigation confirmed that an intimidating culture existed and, disturbingly, highlighted that 80% of these staff had been physically sick, on at least one occasion, before going to work on the Birthing Unit, because of the fear of going to work. The fear experienced by staff of speaking up when interviewed cannot be underestimated and support was made available to staff following their interview.

Three senior midwives were identified as the main persons by almost all staff interviewed, with some of the senior midwives being thought to 'role-model' these individuals, culminating in a culture of fear and intimidation. The HOM was presented with the findings of the investigation; the names of the identified persons remained confidential throughout the process. A decision was made that the culture on the birthing unit had 'expected' midwives to behave in this way, for many years, under a previous management style, but this was no longer acceptable. Therefore, the three midwives were met individually, with their union representatives, and it was explained to them that disrespectful behaviour was no longer acceptable, a line was drawn in the sand, and they were informed that if incidents occurred in the future, the disciplinary procedure would be initiated. The three midwives were moved from the birthing unit and offered individual counselling and support.

A decision was made in consultation with human resources, and the maternity unit General Manager for the HOM to design and run workshops, which every member of staff was expected and rostered alphabetically to attend. The intention of the workshops was to identify and raise awareness of what constitutes bullying behaviour, the psychological, physiological and behavioural harm caused and strategies for dealing with it. The workshops emphasised that a zero tolerance to disrespectful behaviour had been implemented and that all allegations of bullying would be taken extremely seriously. The culture slowly improved, and midwives' confidence began to increase. Two years later, there was a waiting list of midwives to join the maternity unit, together with a big reduction in numbers of midwives leaving, reduced sickness rates and complaints.

<table>
<tr><td>

Make disrespectful and bullying behaviour unacceptable by implementing a zero-tolerance policy

All allegations of unacceptable behaviour to be treated seriously by the whole management/leadership team.

Co-create a set of acceptable and unacceptable behaviours with all maternity and neonatal staff and hold everyone accountable for upholding them

Create credibility and confidence by making your own views of unacceptable behaviour known and act immediately when 'someone crosses the line'

When allegations are made ensure psychological safety is maintained within the area

Treat both the person making the allegation and the person identified as displaying disrespectful behaviour with compassion and ensure emotional support is available for both.

Advise both parties to seek support, advice and representation from their trade union/professional body

Follow HR advice and follow your organisations policies and guidelines.

</td></tr>
</table>

**Fig. 8.2** Summary of actions towards achieving respectful relationships

Once zero tolerance to unacceptable behaviour is established and staff know you will act, kindness and compassion will gradually become embedded in everyday culture (Fig. 8.2).

### 8.3.2  Achieving Inclusion

Equity, diversity inclusion and belonging (EDIB) are essential to achieving culture change (Smith 2021) and are identified as one of the 'golden threads of change' (OED 2025) woven throughout the book (see Sects. 2.5 and 7.2). Without inclusion, the culture is not compassionate (West 2021). As a reminder, an inclusive culture is one where 'it is psychologically and physically safe for *all* staff, irrespective of their race, gender, sexual or religious orientation, culture, disabilities, learning disabilities, neurodiversity and mental and physical challenges to be the person they are' (Smith 2021, p. 128). All organisations should have an Equal Opportunities policy that is regularly monitored and 'all employers, managers and employees should understand the importance of equality, diversity and inclusion in all areas of work' (ACAS 2025), including the following:

- Recruiting new staff.
- Training and promoting existing staff.
- Equal pay.
- Religious beliefs and practice.
- Dress code.
- Unacceptable behaviour.
- The dismissal of staff.
- Redundancy.
- Different types of leave for parents.
- Flexible working.

As health professionals, we cannot ignore the fact that poor outcomes are higher for Black and Asian women and pregnant people and babies, with maternal mortality three times higher for Black women and two times higher for Asian women, than for a White woman (Felker et al. 2024). Additionally, recent reports have highlighted that racism exists within the NHS (Darzi 2024) and maternity services (CQC 2024; Kirkup 2022); this is reflected in the maternity care women and birthing people receive.

> Communication with women and their families is not always good enough, particularly for those with protected equality characteristics. This affects their ability to consent to treatment and can perpetuate levels of fear and anxiety. (CQC 2024, p. 4)

Racism is reflected in the treatment of staff from ethnic minority backgrounds, with them being less likely to be promoted into senior positions, facing greater barriers to career progression, being more likely to enter former disciplinary process and experience more harassment, bullying and abuse from colleagues, patients and their relatives than their white colleagues (Smith 2021, p. 110). This section makes recommendations and gives examples of *how* compassionate leaders have improved inclusion for staff, women and birthing people and neonates in the maternity and neonatal services they have held responsibility for.

Understand your own unconscious bias; are you aware of and do you understand your own unconscious bias? This is defined by Advisory, Arbitration and Conciliatory Service (ACAS) as

> Having beliefs and views about other people that might not be right or reasonable and includes when a person thinks:
>
> - better of someone because they believe they're alike
> - less of someone because that person is different to them, for example, they might be of a different race, religion or age
>
> This means it is possible to make a decision influenced by false beliefs or assumptions. (ACAS 2025)

Everyone can think in a way that involves unconscious bias, so it is important particularly when managing a service, to be aware that unconscious bias could be affecting everyday behaviour and/or decisions. One of the most common areas to be affected by unconscious bias is recruitment; therefore, when advertising and interviewing, all decisions should be recorded, including reasons for the decisions you make. The importance of understanding the impact of unconscious bias was discussed by most of the compassionate leaders with some speaking about the success of staff training on the subject.

The importance of EDIB training was recognised by The West of England Academic Health Science Network who initiated a pilot entitled Black Maternity Matters (BMM) because unconscious bias, stereotyping and lack of diversity competency were identified as having the potential to result in the provision of health services that disadvantage women from non-White ethnic backgrounds. The pilot was designed to deliver meaningful, actionable improvements with the intention of reducing inequity of outcomes for Black women within maternity systems through a collaborative quality improvement approach. A key component of the pilot was the delivery of cultural competency and diversity fluency education for midwives and Maternity Support Workers (MSW); the aim was to examine unconscious bias and the role of the individual in perpetuating unsafe systems of care for Black women. The BMM pilot demonstrated that anti-racist training improved the knowledge and skills associated with cultural competency in midwives and MSWs. The pilot evaluation demonstrated training participants overestimated their cultural competency at the start of the programme, but by the end had increased their understanding of how racism impacts health inequalities and were able to transfer this knowledge to their work context (Riley et al. 2023). The outcome of the BMM pilot was:

> The style and focus of learning on anti-racism has the potential to cause discomfort but was identified as part of a necessary journey. Creating a focus on the training as anti-racism work has the potential to prioritise the severity of the structural issues of racism and its consequences in healthcare, therefore future iterations of the training should be clearly identified as anti-racism work. This training helped participants improve key understanding, knowledge, and awareness of the impacts of racism, and has the potential to act as a catalyst for change of what can be done differently in healthcare spaces. (Riley et al. 2023)

Ensure that there are robust systems to collect demographic data that can be used to address disparities in outcomes for Black and Asian women (Feeley 2023) and record diversity within the workforce. The CQC in their National Review of Maternity Services 2022–2024 stated: 'We know the inequalities in outcome and additional risks experienced by women from Black and ethnic groups are well documented, yet we found huge differences in the way NHS Trusts collect and use demographic data to try to address those disparities'(CQC 2024, p. 4).

'Compassionate leadership is the means by which we ensure inclusive leadership' (West 2021, p. 132); inclusion and compassionate leadership are 'golden threads' woven throughout the book, both essential to achieving culture change. West (2021) ascertains that where leadership is inclusive, all staff have equal opportunities to progress based on their needs, have opportunities to take on challenging tasks, are provided with support they need and are listened to and respected. When leading people, especially those from minorities who are discriminated against, it is important that as compassionate leaders, we behave consistently. To ensure that you do this, regularly ask yourself the question: am I consistently authentic, honest and open, optimistic, appreciative and compassionate? (West 2021, p. 135). The principles of compassionate leadership can be applied to inclusive leadership as follows:

*Attending*: Listen to all staff equally and consciously seek to have more contact and be present with staff you see as different from yourself. 'Compassionate leadership requires courage and that includes the courage to practise self-awareness in the moment and to identify how our relationships differ amongst those we lead' (West 2021, p. 132). To be genuinely 'present' and attentive, especially when there are so many conflicting priorities can be difficult, but to 'to slow down, be present and listen to those we wish to support is a privileged position many of us hold. We can use this positively and productively to work collaboratively and make long lasting changes. Overriding the desire to fix, slow down, *see* the person and create the space for change to happen is something many of us have to learn to do'. (Smith 2021, p. 113). When attending within a team meeting, or forum, it is important to give everyone an opportunity to speak, to be heard and to ensure that their contribution is respected by all present.

*Understanding* of who is behind the voice, without making assumptions, about the person and the barriers that many people face. When team leaders take the time to fully understand the diversity within the team they lead, it is more likely the team will role-model this behaviour and become able to understand and respect each other's contribution.

*Empathy*: Always demonstrate that you have understood the suffering the person has experienced because of having been treated differently or subjected to unacceptable behaviour because of their difference.

*Helping* is fundamental to being an inclusive leader; it means we help, not merely listen, understand and empathise. West (2021, p. 134) gives an example of helping by explaining that women and those from minority ethnic groups are known to be less likely to be given challenging assignments. This deprives them of growth opportunities, skill development and valuable experience; therefore, compassionate leaders ensure that those who are likely to be victims of discrimination are especially offered challenging opportunities also providing the necessary support to ensure successful completion of these challenges. Helping means to remove obstacles and provide resources to enable staff to do their jobs effectively, for example, a neurodivergent member of staff may not be comfortable working in a loud, busy, antenatal clinic environment, but may be comfortable as a theatre recovery midwife or working in a high dependency unit. Helping includes ensuring all staff receive high-quality, continually improving, compassionate support, including coaching, to enable them to thrive in their roles.

Speak up if you see unfairness and/or discrimination in maternity or neonatal practice or any other area of the service; it is important that you find a way to speak up. Challenging disrespectful and bullying behaviour and what to do if you are unable to challenge it has been discussed (see Sect. 8.2); the same principles apply in challenging unconscious bias and racism. This takes courage, but as a manager, there is a responsibility, and in cases of racism, harassment and discrimination, a legal requirement to act. When a manager fails to act on racism, unmanaged bias, offensive behaviour and all concerns regarding unfair or discriminatory behaviour, or practices, it must be taken seriously by the senior management team of the organisation. The main reason for speaking up and giving feedback should be to help someone to understand the *impact* their behaviour has had. It is also important to give feedback when someone has been inclusive in their behaviour and/or practice which has had a positive impact. Sometimes, it may be necessary to highlight a behaviour that has had a negative impact, even if unintended. When there is a negative *impact,* this may not have been the person's *intention,* which may have been different from the *impact* they caused; therefore, it is important to be compassionate to the person and remain non-judgemental.

> All staff should have training in how to intervene when they observe discrimination, incivility, sexism or racism towards colleagues, all staff should be inclusion allies and champions of equity, equality, positive diversity and inclusion. (West 2021, p. 140)

**Box 8.3 Vignette: Caring Dimensions: One Approach to Achieving Inclusion**
Ivy, a DOM of a large inner-city maternity service, became concerned about an increase in the number of complaints from women and birthing people from Black and Asian women; then, she received one distressing complaint from a person who did not speak English. Added to this, there was an increase in the number of allegations of bullying and increasing sickness amongst the staff. Ivy decided to hold an extraordinary meeting of, at that time, the Maternity Services Liaison Committee (MSLC), whose membership consisted of service users who had had experience of maternity and neonatal care, Ivy as HOM and doctors, midwives and neonatal nurses from all areas of the service; the meeting was chaired by a service user. There was much debate, and it was finally agreed to:

- Create a project group with a term of reference that would be agreed and overseen by the MSLC
- Agree on five of the most serious complaints and convert them into a scenario with a script
- Invite each of the families who had sent the five complaints into the NHS Trust to become involved with creating a scenario and permission was sought from them all to video the scenarios

One of the partners was very keen to be involved and volunteered to join the project group, and he also volunteered to video the scenarios. The project was named 'Caring Dimensions' and a project leader was appointed for two days per week to coordinate the project. Caring Dimensions was publicised throughout the unit and received a lot of interest with several staff volunteering as 'actors'. The five scenarios originating from the complaints and one allegation of bullying involved re-creating care received from a Black woman and birthing person, an Asian woman and birthing person, a Black partner, and a person with disabilities who used a wheelchair, and the fifth scenario was about a midwife who had been bullied. The five scenarios were filmed by the partner, with excellent results, and they were viewed and approved by the complainants before being released for education and training purposes. Following this, all doctors (including consultants), midwives, nurses and maternity care assistants were rostered to attend a raising awareness training

(continued)

**Box 8.3** (continued)

session. The sessions began by giving the context that had led to the videos' creation, the videos were then shown and discussion followed about how care could have been given differently in the four care scenarios and how the midwife could have been treated differently in the bullying scenario. The debates following the showing of the videos were always lively with much discussion and engagement from the staff, with a marked reduction in the number of complaints received from Black and Asian women and allegations of bullying received from staff (Fig. 8.3).

---

Understand your own unconscious bias and the importance of self-awareness

Be aware of the impact of unconscious bias, harassment, victimisation and racism on all areas of the service, including poor outcomes for Black and Asian women and birthing people and on the psychological safety of the staff.

Be aware of your organisation's Equal Opportunity policy and how it is monitored

Ensure there is no opportunity for unconscious bias, within the recruitment process and ensure all decisions are recorded

Ensure there are systems to collect demographic data that can be used to address disparities in outcomes for Black and Asian women and that records diversity within the workforce

Arrange EDI education and training for all staff, for anti-racism, unconscious bias and training in how to intervene when they observe discrimination, incivility, sexism or racism towards colleagues

Always speak up and manage offensive behaviour, unconscious bias, harassment, victimisation and racism and all concerns regarding unfair or discriminatory behaviour or practices.

Ensure you always practice the four qualities of compassionate leadership; attending, understanding, empathy and helping to *all* staff.

---

**Fig. 8.3** Summary of actions towards achieving inclusion

### 8.3.3 Achieving a Coaching Mindset

Embracing a coaching mindset can become a powerful tool to enable positive cultures to grow and develop (see Sect. 5.5). All compassionate leaders identified coaching and developing a coaching mindset as essential to culture change, with some having successfully implemented a coaching mindset within their service. Additionally, coaching has been identified within this book as a 'golden thread of change' (OED 2025) because it has the potential and strength to weave all other factors together to underpin the philosophy of staff supporting and nurturing each other. The importance of listening attentively has previously been discussed and identified as a coaching skill by Helen Rogers and Denise Linay (see Sect. 5.2). If maternity and neonatal units successfully develop a coaching mindset, listening and empathy would be embedded into their culture, aligning with three of the four principles of compassion and compassionate leadership. A compassionate leader's role is to listen to understand someone's pain, demonstrate empathy and help by taking steps to alleviate it. However, a coach's role includes listening to understand and empathy, but does not include helping; it is to support the coachee to find their own solution.

Improving quality of care and experience for women and birthing people and all staff, the CQC (2024) identified significant concerns, highlighted in their National Review of Maternity Services in England Report 2022–2024 regarding communicating, engaging with and listening to women (CQC 2024, p. 7). These concerns were also highlighted by Donna Ockenden in the Independent Maternity Review (2022), recommending that maternity services ensure women are listened to and future CQC inspections assess whether women's voices are truly heard (Independent Maternity Review 2022, p. 27). If a coaching mindset was implemented across all maternity units, 'listening to understand' both women and birthing people and staff would occur naturally, becoming the catalyst to transform negative cultures.

How to embrace a coaching mindset as an individual has previously been detailed in depth by Denise and Helen (see Sect. 5.5), by focusing and exploring the skills required for a coaching conversation; as a reminder these are as follows:

1. Listening to Understand.
2. Questioning.
3. Playback.
4. Feedback.
5. The use of silence.
6. Empathy.

A detailed explanation of each skill is given with exercises and case studies to illustrate points. All six counselling skills are complementary and essential to developing a compassionate culture, particularly *listening to understand* (see Sect. 5.5.1) and *empathy* (see Sect. 5.5.5).

The benefits of coaching for staff within a healthcare setting cannot be underestimated (see Sect. 5.12). As a leader aspiring to transform a negative culture, it will be important to encourage all staff to develop a coaching mindset; this is possible to be achieved through the planned implementation of a coaching programme. The details of who will be the first to receive coaching, how many individuals will be coached at one time and how many sessions each person receives will require discussion and agreement. Whom you decide to include in your first tranche will send a message to staff regarding who is considered to be the 'most important'; therefore, this decision and how it is communicated are an important one. When deciding on this point, remember the importance of inclusion and avoiding unconscious bias. The coaching plan should be agreed, supported and communicated by all leaders and managers. A business case will be required to obtain funding for the cost of providing coaching, together with any staff backfill that may be required. To achieve this, demonstrate how staffing costs can be reduced through reducing staff sickness and attrition, including recruitment costs. A reduction in the number of allegations of harassment and bullying should occur, clinical incidents should reduce because of improved physiological safety with less complaints and improved experience for women and birthing people as staff develop and put coaching skills into action.

Decide on the group of staff to be the first to be coached, how many can receive coaching at any one time and how many sessions they can have.

Write a business plan, including the financial costs and benefits, of rolling out a coaching programme.

Investigate 'in-house' coaching or the purchase of coaching sessions, ensuring the provider is accredited and reputable.

Once a coaching programme is established actively encourage all staff to develop a coaching mindset

Once underway, evaluate the impact of the coaching programme on both staff and women and birthing people

**Fig. 8.4** Summary of actions towards achieving a coaching mindset

The NHS Leadership Academy state on their web page (NHS Leadership Academy 2025b) (see Sect. 5.12), that coaching is available for all NHS professions in England, with contact e-mail addresses provided (NHS Leadership Academy 2025a). There are NHS Leadership development programmes in all UK countries, some of which provide individual coaching as part of the course, explored further in Chap. 8 (see Sect. 8.3.5). Coaching may be provided within your NHS Trust, or you may need to purchase/access coaching sessions from a different provider; in this case, to use an accredited coach is very important (see Sect. 5.14). Once a plan to provide coaching for staff is established and underway a ripple effect may occur (see Sect. 5.13), resulting in all staff beginning to develop coaching skills, with a coaching mindset eventually becoming the *way of thinking* (Whitmore 2009), integrated into everyday interactions between all staff and colleagues and women and birthing people. When the coaching programme is well underway, an evaluation should be undertaken using quantitative data regarding numbers of complaints, allegations of bullying and harassment and staff sickness rates and qualitative data looking at staff and women and birthing people's experience (Fig. 8.4).

## 8.3.4 Achieving Values-Based Education (VBE) and Improving Student Experience

The importance of a values-based curriculum is explored in depth in the publication *The University of Southampton Midwifery Values Based Enquiry Journey* (Kitson-Reynolds 2020), with all resources for the VBE curriculum available in Chap. 10 of *A Concise Guide to Continuity of Care in Midwifery* (Kitson-Reynolds and Ashforth 2022). VBE has been discussed by Ellen Kitson-Reynolds and Marie Naish (see Sect. 4.4), where the VBE activity is described as 'a spiral development whereby the students expand their knowledge and explore their 'selves' alongside reflecting on their personal values and beliefs and those they come into contact with. The humanised philosophy is paramount and a constant throughout the curriculum design and delivery' (see Sect. 4.4). The first of the eight yearly VBE activities occurs within fresher's week and involves the students introducing and speaking about themselves (Kitson-Reynolds and Ashforth 2022, p. 149). Following this, ground rules are discussed and agreed by the cohort; being kind to each other is always suggested and supported. This proves invaluable throughout the three-year programme because when reinforcing respectful relationships, students who break this rule can be held to account.

To achieve an improved student experience, treat *all* students with kindness and compassion, and have awareness of your own unconscious bias; each student arrives with their own 'story' and experience, listen to and validate their experiences to ensure that they feel valued and heard as an individual.

> Students want to feel like they will be good midwives, which will be achieved with positive attitudes and behaviours towards them from senior staff during clinical placements. Staff involved with the care of women and newborns should ensure they show students civility and patience while teaching and supporting them. Understanding the level of knowledge that students possess can make it simpler for staff to recognise what each student may or may not have been exposed to. (McNeil and Kitson-Reynolds 2024, p. 1)

To treat students with compassion can be achieved through applying the principles of compassion: attending, understanding, empathising and helping (West et al. 2017). An example of how this can be achieved is demonstrated below:

> **Box 8.4 Vignette: An Example of Supporting a Student Using the Four Principles of Compassionate Leadership**
>
> Amelia, a student midwife went to Terry, her personal tutor, upset and demoralised, because she believed her previous experience and knowledge, as an intensive care unit (ICU) nurse, was being completely discounted whilst she was in clinical practice. Amelia had been a senior ICU nurse for several years before deciding to undertake her midwifery training. Terry was able to apply the four compassionate leadership principles as follows:
>
> *Attend* by listening to Amelia's experience of how she believed her previous level of knowledge and experience was not understood and consequently was being completely discounted.
>
> *Understand* through understanding what Amelia's previous knowledge and experience actually were and how they could be applied to caring for women and birthing people.
>
> *Empathise* by demonstrating that he understood how discounting this level of knowledge and experience made Amelia feel.
>
> *Help* by speaking to Amelia's supervisors and assessors, with her permission, to help them understand how discounting this knowledge and experience made Amelia feel.

Once compassionate cultures are achieved and students feel valued, they will retain their passion and joy of midwifery and are much more likely to continue their midwifery journey after qualification. 'It [compassion] can lead to people experiencing more positive emotions such as gratitude, pride, and inspiration, and can lead to upward emotional spirals that can enhance emotional well-being' (West 2021, p. 66). As with NHS Trusts, it is essential that universities engage compassionate leaders who ensure that all students, from their first contact via the admissions process to the presentation of their final award, are treated compassionately and that we positively embrace difference with true inclusion demonstrated throughout the whole programme.

Psychological safety is as important for a student within an academic setting, as it is within an NHS Trust; as clinical and academic staff, it is our responsibility to ensure that students feel psychologically safe in different environments. Achieving respectful relationships has been previously discussed (see Sect. 8.3.1) with the same principles applying within a university setting; we need to establish a zero tolerance to disrespectful behaviours and challenge all unacceptable behaviour. All allegations of bullying should be taken seriously; these can include allegations between.

- A student and a member of staff on their clinical placement, for example, a supervisor, assessor, a health professional or a healthcare assistant (HCA).
- A student and a member of the university teaching team, including their personal tutor.
- A student and a student from the same or different cohort.
- Two members of the university teaching team, in which case, the two members of university staff will require support and university human resource (HR) policies will apply.

Once an allegation has been made, follow advice given previously (see Sect. 8.3.1) by using the attending, understanding, empathy and helping principles of compassionate leadership (West et al. 2017). All students should be made aware of available support (see Sects. 4.2 and 8.2) and be encouraged to access it when necessary. By having regular meetings with their allocated students, personal tutors will be able to assess the students' well-being. There is evidence that when students develop compassionate care for themselves and others, this may play a significant role in helping them to face the rigours of education and clinical practice during their degree programme (Beaumont et al. 2016). One way of developing and maintaining psychological safety is to implement Schwartz Rounds, previously described (See Sect. 6.1) as a 'non-judgmental way to provide support to all, reinforcing our values, reminding us why we chose our profession and restoring commitment to compassionate care' (Lown and Manning 2010; Goodrich 2012).

Of students across the UK, 19% are disabled and many find it hard to be heard within their universities (Disabled Students UK 2023). The Disabled Students UK reported in their Insights Access Report 2023 that 1372 disabled students completed a survey questionnaire to measure their experience against six criteria, the criteria together with the measuring criteria in italics and the average results for the UK are detailed below:

1. Universal design—Disabled Students should be greeted by an environment, practices and policies designed with accessibility in mind. *Measured by students having recorded lectures: 61%.*
2. An inclusive culture—Disabled students should experience a positive culture at their institution, which promotes inclusion, belonging and a healthy approach to productivity. *Measured by being made to feel unwelcome because of disability: 26%.*
3. A barrier-free path to support—Disabled students should not have to go through a process that is so difficult that it puts them at a disadvantage in order to receive individualised adjustments. *Measured by being provided with enough information about different adjustments that could help them: 45%.*
4. Sufficient adjustments—Disabled students should receive all reasonable adjustments needed to enable them to access their degree on equal terms with their non-disabled peers. *Measured by all adjustments being provided: 36%.*
5. Somewhere to turn—Disabled students should have a person or place to go to within their institution to effectively resolve accessibility issues. *Measured by having a person or place to go to within their institution to effectively resolve accessibility issues: 59%.*
6. Equal opportunities—Disabled students should be provided with the same non-academic opportunities from their institution as their non-disabled peers. *Measured by feeling part of the community at their university: 42%.*

Although the results varied greatly between universities, some were concerning, for example, only 36% of students with disabilities had received all their reasonable adjustments. The students were asked what would make the most difference and the answer was 'to be listened to' (Disabled Students UK 2023); 'listening' will be achieved if the qualities of compassionate leadership: attending, understanding, empathy and helping (West et al. 2017) are applied to all transactions with students. Before their first clinical placement, the needs of disabled students will require discussion between university and clinical placement staff; especially when reasonable adjustments are required, the student may need NHS Trust occupational health referral when there are concerns about difficulties in undertaking the duties required for the role.

A recommendation to consider is the implementation of an 'Autism Friendly' curriculum, which considers and understands the needs of neurodiverse students, clinical colleagues, other clinicians and women and birthing people. Students who enter university with undiagnosed autism spectrum disorder (ASD) and attention-deficit hyperactivity disorder (ADHD) face difficulties because they often require rapid access to diagnostic services, medical care including psychoeducation and medication, and educational support (Sedgewick-Müller 2024). However, waiting lists for ASD and ADHD diagnosis and support are often longer than the duration of an undergraduate degree. In these circumstances, it is important to direct the student to the Disability and Inclusion Teams, as soon as possible after entry, because reasonable adjustments, educational and personal tutor support, and Disabled Students'

Ensure the four qualities of compassionate leadership; attending, understanding, empathy and helping (West et al 2017) are applied when interacting with students.

Ensure admissions procedures, curricula and assessments are inclusive and do not put anyone at a disadvantage.

Implement Schwartz Rounds for students in universities.

Ensure all students are aware of available support and how to access it.

Encourage students to practice compassion towards themselves and others

Consider implementing an 'Autism Friendly' curriculum

Be aware of students with disabilities, 'listen' to them, and review their reasonable adjustments regularly with the student and the university disability and inclusion teams.

University and clinical staff should work together to ensure students with disabilities are supported in both academic and clinical settings. The students should be referred to NHS Trusts occupational health if there are concerns about their ability to carry out the required duties of the role.

**Fig. 8.5** Summary of actions towards achieving values-based education and improving student experience

Allowance (DSA) can promote positive learning experiences for students with ASD and ADHD. Students with ASD and ADHD identified through university are more likely to receive a non-medical diagnosis, which enables reasonable adjustments to be put in place and an application for DSA to be supported (Sedgewick-Müller 2024) (Fig. 8.5).

## 8.3.5　Achieving Culture Change Through Compassionate Leadership

Compassionate leadership examples (see Chap. 7) have previously been given of how leaders demonstrate compassionate leadership and how the principles of attending, understanding, empathy and helping (West et al. 2017) can be applied to situations where culture change is required (see Sect. 7.2.3). The case study below describes how a compassionate leader (pseudonym Vera) achieved the implementation of compassionate models of midwifery, physiological safety, inclusion and respectful relationships by changing a hierarchical, depersonalised and negative culture to a compassionate, kind and psychologically safe culture. Vera used the principles of compassionate leadership of attending, understanding, empathy and helping (West et al. 2017) and Social Capital theory, described by the Institute for Social Capital (2025) as:

> Fundamentally, it denotes the innate ability, capacity, and potential of individuals to engage in collaborative, positive interactions and collective efforts. At its essence, Social Capital is rooted in the understanding that social relationships are invaluable assets, capable of catalysing positive and productive actions while curbing counterproductive and negative behaviors. (Institute for Social Capital 2025)

Vera believed that combining the principles of compassionate leadership with Social Capital theory would be transformational.

**Box 8.5 Case study: Achieving Culture Change**

Vera was the HOM responsible for five standalone maternity units in a rural setting. She had inherited a maternity service culture that was hierarchical, depersonalised and psychologically unsafe. Vera was aware that an inclusive, compassionate model of midwifery was required across the service, and she knew that it was important for the midwives to 'own' and agree the new model. Firstly, in line with Social Capital theory, Vera started to develop networks across the service; one of the networks that would prove invaluable was to develop a Band 7 network through the development of a leadership course for all Band 7 midwives. By meeting and learning about each together, a respectful, supportive network developed that continued to meet after the course had finished. The leadership course included individual coaching, which was powerful and transformational in achieving the culture change required. Vera also made a business case to her NHS Trust Board for coaching for all professional staff and eventually received funding for this.

Having prepared the staff with training and development, the next step was arranging to consult with users of the service, to determine how women and birthing people felt about the current service and what type of service they wanted. To do this, Vera arranged forums with as many women and birthing people and partners as possible and midwives, in each of the five units, and sent out a questionnaire to all women and birthing people. Four questions were asked to begin the discussion:

Did you feel safe?
Did you feel welcome?
Did you have someone with you?
Did you have someone who could explain things in a way you could understand?

The response and points raised in the discussion were used to inform the development of a new model of midwifery care. Vera's next step was to develop a vision for the new model of care and determine the values that everyone would be expected to uphold. Workshops and forums were organised, a vision and values were agreed and consulted upon, with a copy sent to *all* staff within the service. Every midwife contributed to the development of the new model of care; it was then consulted on and agreement reached with the midwives who were represented by the RCM. Regular short meetings were held for staff within each of the five units and separate meetings for the team leads across all five units. The ground rules for the meetings were:

*(continued)*

> **Box 8.5** (continued)
>
> The values were said aloud at the start of each meeting.
> Everyone was able to have conversations about behaviours.
> Questions asked were always open and no one was 'picked on'.
> Clinical supervision occurred when necessary and everyone was encouraged
>   to speak about clinical situations they may have found difficult.
> Every midwife was designated a 'champion' for one aspect of practice.
> Everyone was encouraged to challenge disrespectful behaviour.
>
> Staff began to feel safe and supported and as a result felt able to challenge disrespectful behaviour, were able to make decisions and practise autonomously, believing that they would be supported by colleagues and managers.

Leadership programmes were identified by all leaders as important for developing aspiring leaders; there are several courses available, and it is important to select the right ones that match the values of your organisation. Below are a few of the programmes available and all were spoken recommended by at least one compassionate leader:

- The All-Wales Midwifery Leadership and Development Programme (MLDG) a joint Welsh Government and RCM Wales initiative (see Sect. 5.6) includes coaching for its participants.
- NHS Education Scotland (2025)—Leading for the Future programme that includes coaching (NHS Education for Scotland 2025).
- NHS England—Culture and Leadership course that includes coaching and provided for the senior management team for every NHS Trust in England that has maternity services (NHS England 2025).
- NHS Leadership Academy-run leadership courses (NHS Leadership Academy 2025a).

*Consider external support* to work with you to achieve culture change; this can be for a maternity and/or neonatal department or for an entire NHS Trust or organisation. If you decide to invest in support to help you change your working culture, 'A Kind Life' is an example of a company with a good reputation, which has achieved excellent results, all available on their website (A Kind Life 2024). It is important to find a company whose approach aligns with the attributes of compassionate leadership and who has achieved measurable results. A Kind Life provides a range of education and training including large-scale workshops and leadership development as well as i-learning modules.

**Advice from Compassionate Leaders to Achieve Culture Change** The following points were given by leaders who have achieved positive culture change within maternity services:

- My first thoughts are always 'what do I need to do to bring people with me?'
- You need to have trusted people that you can talk to.
- The staff had been micro-managed; I had to make them believe I trusted them.
- You can't do it on your own, I had to find allies in the team to work with to identify solutions.
- To have co-created vision and values is important with *everyone* having a voice in creating them.
- Learn as you go, you can't expect to go in and be perfect.
- In time, you have to have an opinion, staff expect that.
- When you know that it's going to be tough, choose 'low hanging fruit' to get started.
- Culture is constantly evolving; you never start with A and end up at B.
- The important thing is to create a team around you, each with different skills.
- Create opportunities to bring out the best in people.
- Allow people to do what they are good at.
- When dealing with conflict, dignity is essential.
- Respect student's previous knowledge and experience.
- It's all down to humanity.
- You need so much courage.
- Developing caring networks is essential.
- Negotiation and collaboration are essential skills.
- Sometimes, leadership has to happen at the right point in your life.
- The culture of the NHS, including racism, impacts Black and Asian women and staff.
- Ask: do you know what your colleagues do?
- We have appointed staff in posts with a view to helping to achieve culture change, for example, the NHSE-funded recruitment and retention midwives.
- Succession planning is very important to maintain the level of change achieved (Fig. 8.6).

<table>
<tr><td>Ensure the four qualities of compassionate leadership; attending, understanding, empathy and helping (West et al 2017) are applied from the beginning to end of the culture change process</td></tr>
<tr><td>Investigate Leadership Programmes for different cohorts of staff, both internally and externally, that use the principles of compassionate leadership</td></tr>
<tr><td>Invest in a programme of coaching for staff; write a business case to obtain funding (see Sect 8.3.3)</td></tr>
<tr><td>Co-create a vision and values with all grades of staff and professions, including users of the service. Once the values are agreed and communicated, hold all staff accountable to uphold them.</td></tr>
<tr><td>Consider appointing midwives into posts with the intention of assisting culture change (Feeley and Stacey, 2024)</td></tr>
<tr><td>Ensure that succession planning is a priority to maintain the culture change achieved</td></tr>
</table>

**Fig. 8.6** Summary of actions towards achieving culture change through compassionate leadership

## 8.3.6 Implementing Compassionate Models of Care

The Kings Fund ABC framework of core work needs (West et al. 2020; West 2021) encapsulates all that has been recommended within this book and is recommended as a clear, compassionate model possible to align with a midwifery model of care.

> Meeting people's core needs at work ensures they have high levels of intrinsic motivation and high levels of well-being. They are likely to be highly motivated and to find their work joyful rather than depleting and damaging. (West 2021, p. 119)

The 'ABC of nurses' and midwives' core work needs model' is detailed in West et al.'s (2020) report entitled *The courage of compassion: supporting nurses and midwives to deliver high quality care*. The model is derived from the authors' qualitative and quantitative research to explore the causes and consequences of poor mental health and well-being among nurses and midwives, following the COVID-19 pandemic. The research established an ABC of core work needs (West et al. 2020):

- *Autonomy and control*—the need to have control over our work lives and to act consistently with our work life and values.
- *Belonging*—the need to be connected to, cared for. And caring of others around us in the workplace and you feel valued, respected and supported.
- *Contribution and competence*—the need to experience effectiveness and deliver valued outcomes such as high-quality care.

West (2021, p. 121–122) details the implementation of the ABC model as follows:

**Autonomy and Control**

1. Authority, empowerment and influence: Influence over decisions about how care is structured and delivered, ways of working and organisational culture.
   - Introduce mechanisms for staff to shape the cultures and processes of their organisations and influence decisions about how care is structured and delivered.
2. Justice and fairness: Equity, physiological safety, positive diversity and universal inclusion.
   - Nurture and sustain just, fair and psychologically safe cultures and ensure equity proactive and positive approaches to diversity and universal inclusion.
3. Work conditions and work schedules: Resources, time and permission to properly rest, eat and drink, and to work safely, flexibly and effectively.
   - Introduce minimum standards for facilities and working conditions for staff.

**Belonging**

4. Teamworking: Effectively functioning, stable teams with role clarity and shared objectives, one of which is team member well-being.
   - Develop and support effective multidisciplinary team working for all staff across health and social care.
5. Culture and leadership: Nurturing cultures and compassionate leadership enabling high-quality, continually improving and compassionate patient care and staff support.
   - Ensure that health and social care environments have compassionate leadership and nurturing cultures that enable both care and staff support to be high-quality, continually improving and compassionate.

**Contribution and Confidence**

6. Workload: Work demands at levels that enable the sustainable delivery of safe, compassionate care and staff well-being.
   - Tackle chronic excessive work demands on staff, which exceed their capacity to sustainably lead and deliver safe, high-quality care and which damage their health and well-being.
7. Management and supervision: The support, professional reflection and supervision to enable staff to thrive in their work.
   - Ensure that all staff have the effective support, professional reflection, mentorship and supervision needed to thrive in their roles.
8. Education, learning and development: Flexible, high-quality development opportunities that promote continuing growth and development for all.
   - Ensure that right systems, frameworks and processes are in place for learning, education and development throughout people's careers. These should promote fair and equitable outcomes.

It is possible to implement a midwifery model of care that builds upon the West et al.'s (2020) ABC framework of core work needs; an example of this is the ASSET model, developed from research findings to demonstrate that midwives are an asset for both women and birthing people and employers (Feeley 2023, p88). The ASSET model mirrors the Kings Fund ABC framework of core work needs, complementing and extending it for midwives, because it is 'rooted in supporting the needs of midwives to practice autonomously' (Feeley 2023, p. 89).

*The New Zealand (NZ) Lead Maternity Carer (LMC) model of care* (Guilliland and Pairman 1994) is internationally acclaimed, has existed for 30 years and provides opportunities for midwives to practise in a way they are philosophically aligned to. The model consists of LMC midwives taking a caseload and providing continuity of care to all women and birthing people booked with them. McAra-Couper et al. (2014) cite Guilliland and Pairman (1994) in describing the LMC model of care as 'philosophically based on the woman-midwife relationship being one of partnership. This relationship is one of reciprocity and trust and has long informed the midwife-woman relationship in NZ'. The LMC model enables a large majority of NZ women and birthing people to have midwifery-led continuity of care throughout the antenatal, labour and postnatal periods. NZ maternity services integrate primary, secondary and tertiary services with its midwives choosing to practise as an LMC or to be employed by the District Health Boards as 'core midwives'. As core midwives, they usually work shifts and care for women who are admitted with complex needs, and they provide support for the LMCs. LMCs are contracted directly to the Ministry of Health and are paid directly by them, meaning they are not obligated to provide maternity care to a particular maternity service (for example, they cannot be required to staff labour wards in time of staff shortages). The LMCs have universal right of access to hospitals for midwives, women and babies when specialist obstetric care is required.

Before a midwifery student enters university, they will know the model of care they will practise within once qualified, no matter where they work in NZ (O'Brien 2022). Once qualified, they must choose between becoming an LMC midwife providing continuity of care, including on-calls, or be employed in a maternity unit as a core midwife. This choice not only means a midwife can work in a way she is fundamentally aligned to but also means when life circumstances change, the midwife can, for example, reduce hours by reducing her caseload, or if she is not able to work on-calls, she can change the way in which she works by joining the core staff in a maternity unit.

McAra-Couper et al. (2014) undertook qualitative, descriptive research by interviewing eleven LMC on-call midwives, with experience ranging from eight to twenty years, to answer the research question 'What sustains midwives in LMC practice?' The findings were as follows:

> The findings show that the primary factor that sustains them is the joy experienced in the reciprocal relationship formed when LMC midwives work in partnership with women and their families/ whanau. The joy of midwifery practice is reflected in a passion for 'being with' women and families, supporting and empowering them through their childbirth experiences and to have the birth they aspire to. The joy underpins the sustainability of midwives in LMC practice. (McAra-Couper et al. 2014)
> This study demonstrated that when midwives are able to work in ways they are fundamentally aligned to, the joy of birth sustains them in practice.

It is recommended that wherever possible, midwives are encouraged and enabled to practise in roles that align with their philosophy of care (see Sect. 2.6); 'it would seem that tackling a bullying culture will require attention to the fundamental ideological underpinnings of practice addressing any paradoxes that exist' (Hunter 2005, p. 264). Feeley and Stacey (2024, p. 2) suggest that there is 'an ongoing tension between midwives' values and expectations of the profession and the actual experience of the role itself'. Additionally, when midwives are fundamentally misaligned to the way in which they practise, their well-being can be impacted (see Sects. 2.6 and 3.3.2) (Maben et al. 2023) and, in some cases, their mental health (Smith 2021). The midwifery model of care often determines whether midwives and student midwives remain in the midwifery profession (Curtis et al. 2006; RCM 2016).

It is recommended to use the principles of compassionate leadership of attending, understanding, empathy and helping (West et al. 2017) to know and understand your staff, including a knowledge of protected characteristics (see Sect. 2.7.6), making it possible to appoint/promote them into roles that align with their philosophy of care. All midwives are philosophically aligned to different models of care (Hunter 2004; Feeley 2023) and ways of working, just as women and birthing people have differing needs; for example, some request a caesarean section for no clinical reason and some request a home birth when they have complications of pregnancy. It is crucial, if culture change is to be achieved, for all midwives, managers and leaders to understand and accept this so that conflict can be avoided as much as possible. Everyone should be valued for their contribution; a community midwife practising in a home birth team is as important as a midwife coordinating a labour ward in a tertiary referral maternity unit, as an MCA working on the postnatal ward, as the HOM. To ask a midwife to work in a way they are misaligned to, especially without notice, will cause stress and anxiety; for example, to call in a community midwife at short notice to staff a high-risk labour ward with no preparation and then for her to be criticised is at best stressful and at worse, traumatic. An understanding of this principle will explain why some midwives felt fear and threatened when it looked as if they would be required to hold a caseload, following the recommendations of the Changing Childbirth report (DH 1993) and much later, the 'Better Births' report (NHS England 2016), resulting in the reaction to resist implementation as strongly as possible.

**Compassionate Ways of Working**  It is not only practising in ways that midwives are misaligned to that causes conflict; this may also occur when staff have no autonomy over the way in which they work, for example, shift patterns, length and/or the requirement to be on-call. Within maternity units, there is often debate about how 'accommodating' managers should be when agreeing shift patterns, for example, allowing midwives to work 'fixed' shifts or to not work night duty for a period of time. It is important to practise compassionate leadership when deciding on staff ways of working; all requests should be listened to and considered individually, especially the reasons for each request, which could be for physical or mental health reasons, or for reasons related to protected characteristics (see Sect. 2.7.6). From experience, when staff are supported through a personal crisis, they will be loyal to the maternity unit, remaining in post, with less sick leave. By implementing the Kings Fund ABC framework of core work needs (West et al. 2020) and the principles of compassionate leadership (West 2021), ways of working will be aligned to the needs of the staff.

*Consultation* is an important step when deciding on and implementing new models of care and ways of working. To avoid misunderstandings along the way, always consult with trade unions/professional bodies from the beginning of the process (Fig. 8.7).

Consider implementing the Kings Fund ABC of core work needs (West et al 2020, West, 2021) as a framework for a compassionate model of care.

Create and implement models of care where midwives can work in ways that are aligned with their philosophy of midwifery care. To achieve this, consider the case study Achieving Culture Change (see Box 8.4) and the ASSET Model (Feeley, 2023)

Use the principles of compassionate leadership to know and understand your staff (including a knowledge of protected characteristics)

Consult with trade unions/professional bodies as soon as possible in the process

Value everyone equally, no matter their role

When implementing new models of care consider the needs of every member of staff,

Use the principles of compassionate leadership when considering individual members of staff ways of working i.e shift patterns

**Fig. 8.7** Summary of actions to implement compassionate models of care

## 8.3.7　Achieving Psychological Safety

Psychological safety is a 'golden thread of change' (OED 2025) running throughout the book critical to achieving positive cultural change (see Chap. 3). Psychological safety will be achieved when the 'golden threads' of compassionate leadership, inclusion, a coaching mindset and respectful relationships are implicit within the maternity culture. The impact on staff when they do not feel physiologically safe has a detrimental effect on the safety of women and birthing people and neonates. Psychological safety enables staff to feel safe to speak out about errors, problems and uncertainties, which will create safer clinical environments for maternity and neonatal staff and for women and birthing people and neonates (see Sects. 3.6 and 7.2.2) (Kirkup 2015, 2022). For staff to report and discuss all clinical incidents and to feel safe to raise concerns, they must trust that the clinical governance processes in place are just and fair. NHS England has published a 'Just culture guide' NHSE (n.d.) that is available for all NHS Trusts to use:

> The fair treatment of staff supports a culture of fairness, openness and learning in the NHS by making staff feel confident to speak up when things go wrong, rather than fearing blame.
>
> Supporting staff to be open about mistakes allows valuable lessons to be learnt so the same errors can be prevented from being repeated. In any organisations or teams where a blame culture is still prevalent, this guide will be a powerful tool in promoting cultural change. (NHSE n.d.)

*Achieving a safe level of staffing* is the most essential factor required to achieve psychological safety and cultural change. Compassionate leaders spoke about how hard it is to achieve safe staffing levels, particularly in times of austerity and when cost savings are mandatory, therefore it is essential to acquire the skills to write robust business cases and to have the confidence to articulate your case to your NHS Trust Board.

Compassionate leaders gave the following advice to midwifery leaders/managers:

- Always know what your full-time equivalent (FTE) numbers of staff are and where they are placed.
- Each 0.1 FTE is important; for example, if a full-time midwife reduces to four days per week, there will be 0.2 FTE released to go towards another post.
- Have a safe, agreed, recommended FTE for each area/department and know how many vacancies you have in each area.
- Establish safe levels of staffing for each ward/department and reach agreement with the staff working in the area (using the principles of compassionate leadership: attending, understanding, empathy, helping [West et al. 2017]) as to what these are.
- Have robust ways of collecting your data regarding vacancy, sickness, maternity/paternity leave rates and know what these are at any one time.
- Have regular meetings with your designated accountant and/or general manager to discuss your staffing budgets.
- If you believe that your FTE numbers of staff are not safe, for example, are below agreed levels of safe staffing, it is essential that you raise this to the highest level of the organisation.
- The staff on shift *must* raise risk forms when staffing is unsafe on their shift, and managers *must* raise the issue, in writing, with their next line of management, all the way up to the NHS Trust Board.
- When unsafe staffing issues are discussed, always ensure that these discussions are recorded, including any decisions reached and actions agreed.

*The importance of achieving psychological safety within teams* has been discussed previously (see Sect. 3.6) and is also a 'golden thread' (OED 2025) running through the book: 'there are clear links between the quality of team working, quality of patient care, patient satisfaction and staff well-being' (West 2021). West (2021, p. 96)) discusses how we create psychological safety within teams which are reflected below:

- Shared visions, values and objectives.
- Reflexivity, innovation and learning.
- Frequent, positive contact.
- Valuing diversity, difference and positive conflict.
- Mutual support, compassion and humility.

*The effectiveness of Schwartz Rounds* has been previously discussed in depth by Emer Kelly (see Chap. 6) and it is recommended that Schwartz Rounds are implemented both in maternity and neonatal units and in universities because they have the potential to provide a non-judgemental way of providing support to all professions, reinforcing our values, reminding us why we chose our profession and restoring commitment to compassionate care. Schwartz Rounds can foster a psychologically safe workplace (Maben et al. 2018) by revealing the person behind the professional and breaking down hierarchies which can enhance staff engagement and increase staff morale. The Point of Care Foundation provides information

---

Compassionate leadership and inclusion are central components to achieving psychological safety

Agree safe levels of staffing with the staff in each area and have robust data collection and reporting mechanisms in place for when staffing levels become unsafe

Ensure clinical governance process are just and fair, consider using the NHSE (nd) Just culture guide.

Consider the team dynamics of each team, looking at ways of nurturing their development

Managers should acquire the skills required to write robust business plans and present them to the Trust Board when necessary

Consider creating and appointing to innovative posts, that have the potential to influence culture change.

Implement Schwartz Rounds with the intention of increasing staff morale and enhancing staff engagement.

---

**Fig. 8.8** Summary of actions to achieve psychological safety

and excellent advice on how to implement Schwartz Rounds (Point of Care Foundation 2015).

The creation of innovative posts that support midwives in practice can be instrumental in achieving psychological safety and positive cultural change. The principle of creating innovative roles was first envisaged by the Department of Health (DH) in its report *Making a Difference: Strengthening the nursing, midwifery and health visiting contribution to health and healthcare* (DH 1999), where it outlined its vision for future consultant nurses' and midwives' roles. The proposed aim of the consultant midwife role was to encourage the development of clinical leadership skills, retain expert clinical skills and to transform maternity services for the improvement of health outcomes for mothers and babies (Wilson et al. 2018). Following the publication of *Making a Difference* (DH 1999), the role of consultant midwife was introduced together with guidance that all consultant midwife roles should encompass four pillars: clinical practice, education, leadership and research (DH 1999). Consultant midwives were initially employed to focus on public health, lead midwifery practice, lead education and training and research, with a few posts created in partnership with universities, providing a link between practice and education with the intention of reducing the practice/education gap. These roles are innovative and transformational in leading culture change, however the opportunities and benefits of employing consultant midwives have been missed by many NHS Trusts across the UK; in 2018, only 84 were identified as being employed by approximately one-third of UK NHS Trusts and Health Boards (Wilson et al. 2018). In their publication, *Where are the consultant midwives?,* Wilson et al. (2018) conclude: 'Given the national imperatives for high-quality maternity care, there needs to be a focus on succession planning and growth of the role of consultant midwives across all organisations'. (Fig. 8.8)

---

## 8.4 Conclusion

The earlier chapters identified the intense pressures that maternity services are currently experiencing: 'Midwives are under unsustainable pressure, and this has been increasing over time' (West et al. 2020). However, there are a few individuals who abuse power; it is clear that if we are to stop disrespectful and bullying behaviours, a cultural change is required that publicises and rigorously adheres to a zero-tolerance approach. We can achieve cultural change by following and implementing the 'golden threads of change' (OED 2025), identified as respectful relationships, inclusion, values-based education, developing a coaching mindset, compassionate leadership, the model of care and psychological safety; all are essential to achieving positive maternity cultures. This final chapter has recommended actions to achieve culture change; some are easy to achieve and others incredibly hard.

The book has spoken directly to anyone who is or has been impacted by disrespectful behaviour, displayed towards them or another member of staff. To these staff members and students, thank you for reading the book, which is a positive first step towards change; the authors hope this book has given you the courage to challenge unacceptable behaviours and the tools to know how to do so. The final question is: 'after reading this book and undertaking the exercises, has your confidence to challenge unacceptable behaviour increased?' Whoever you are, wherever you work, *now* is the time to take that important first small or transformational step towards change. We know there is once again much change on the horizon and many people are currently worried and apprehensive; however, the opportunity is there for us all to create compassionate and kind workplaces if we all work together with courage and respect.

## References

A Kind Life (2024) Kinder Culture with a Kind Life Available at: https://www.akind.life/ (Accessed 28 Feb 2025)

Advisory, Arbitration and Conciliatory Service ACAS (2025) Equality, diversity and inclusion Unconscious bias. Available https://www.acas.org.uk/improving-equality-diversity-and-inclusion/unconscious-bias (accessed 18 Feb 2025)

Aunger J, Maben J, Abrams R, Wright J, Mannion R, Pearson M, Jones A, Westbrook J (2023) Drivers of unprofessional behaviour between staff in acute care hospitals: a realist review. BMC Health Serv Res 23

Baumeister RF, Leary MR (1995) The need to belong: desire for interpersonal attachments as a fundamental human motivation. Psychological Bulletin 117(3); pp. 497–529

Beaumont E, Durkin M, Martin CJH et al (2016) Compassion for others, self-compassion, quality of life and mental well-being measures and their association with compassion fatigue and burnout in student midwives: A quantitative survey. Midwifery 34:239-244. Available: https://doi.org/10.1016/j.midw.2015.11.002 (Accessed 24 Feb 2025)

Capper T 2021 Workplace bullying: The midwifery student experience [Online]. CQ University Australia. Available: https://acquire.cqu.edu.au/articles/thesis/Workplace_bullying_The_midwifery_student_experience/14776482/1/files/28395063.pdf (accessed 26 Jan 2025).

Care Quality Commission (2024) National Review of Maternity Service 2022 – 2024. Available: https://www.cqc.org.uk/publications/maternity-services-2022-2024 (accessed 5 Feb 2025)

Catling C, Reid F, Hunter B (2017) Australian midwives' experiences of their workplace culture. Women and Birth. 30(2):137–145 Available: https://doi.org/10.1016/j.wombi.2016.10.001 (Accessed 25 Feb 2025)

Curtis P, Ball L, Kirkham M (2006). 'Why do midwives leave? (Not) being the kind of midwife you want to be'. British Journal of Midwifery,14 (1 January): 27-29-31 Available https://shura.shu.ac.uk/323/ (accessed 28 Jan 2025)

Darzi, A. (2024) Independent Investigation of the National Health Service in England. Crown Copyright. Available https://www.gov.uk/government/publications/independent-investigation-of-the-nhs-in-england (Accessed 4 Feb 2025)

Department of Health (1993). Changing Childbirth: Report of the Expert Maternity Group Pt.1. London: HMSO

Department of Health (1999) Making a Difference. Strengthening the nursing, midwifery and health visiting contribution to health and healthcare. Available: http://www.nursingleadershiporg.uk/publications/nurstrat.pdf (Accessed 24 Feb 2025)

Disabled Students UK (2023) Access Insight Report 2023. Framework and Baseline. Available: https://disabledstudents.co.uk/wp-content/uploads/2023/11/Disabled-Students-UK_Access-Insights-2023-Report.pdf (Accessed 24 Feb 2025)

Elliott M (2004) The RCM's New President Speaks Out. RCM Midwives Journal 7(6), p. 232.

End Workplace Abuse (2025) Workplace Psychological Safety Act. Available: https://endworkplaceabuse.com/workplace-psychological-safety-act/ (Accessed 4 Feb 2025)

Feeley C, Stacey T (2024) Novel solutions to the midwifery retention crisis in England: an organisational case study of midwives' intentions to leave the profession and the role of retention midwives. Midwifery. Available: https://doi.org/10.1016/j.midw.2024.104152 (accessed 28 Jan 2025)

Feeley C (2023) Skilled Heartfelt midwifery Practice. Safe, Relational Care for Alternative Physiological Births. Springer, Switzerland Available https://doi.org/10.1007/978-3-031-43643-7 (accessed 7 Feb 2025)

Felker A, Patel R, Kotnis R, Kenyon S, Knight M (Eds.) on behalf of MBRRACE-UK. Saving Lives, Improving Mothers' Care Compiled Report – Lessons learned to inform maternity care from the UK and Ireland Confidential Enquiries into Maternal Deaths and Morbidity 2020-22. Oxford: National Perinatal Epidemiology Unit, University of Oxford 2024.

Gillen P, Sinclair M, Kernohan WG (2004) 'A concept analysis of bullying in midwifery'. Evidence Based Midwifery. 2(2):46–51. Available: https://pure.ulster.ac.uk/ws/portalfiles/portal/92266800/scan_e10047419_2021_09_16_15_58_48.pdf (accessed 28 Jan 2025)

Gillan P Sinclair M, Kernohan WG (2008) The nature and manifestations of bullying in midwifery. Belfast: Ulster University. Available: https://pure.ulster.ac.uk/ws/portalfiles/portal/101327391/Gillen_2008_bullying.pdf (accessed 26 Jan 2025)

Gillen P, Sinclair M, Kernohan GW, Begley C (2009) 'Student midwives' experience of bullying. Evidence-Based Midwifery, 7(2):46+. Available: https://link.gale.com/apps/doc/A204894578/HRCA?u=anon~4ec74bf6&sid=googleScholar&xid=08e2bf29 (accessed 27 Jan 2025)

Goodrich J (2012) Supporting hospital staff to provide compassionate care: do Schwartz center rounds work in English hospitals? J R Soc Med. 105(3): 117–22. Available: https://doi.org/10.1258/jrsm.2011.110183 (accessed 4 Feb 2025)

Guilliland K and Pairman S (1994) The Midwifery Partnership – A model for Practice. New Zealand College of Midwives Journal, 5-9.H

Hadikin R, and O'Driscoll M (2000). The bullying culture: cause, effect, harm reduction. Books for Midwives Press, Oxford, England

Hunter B (2004) Conflicting ideologies as a source of emotion work in midwifery. Midwifery 20(3):261-271

Hunter, B. (2005) 'Emotion work and boundary maintenance in hospital-based midwifery', Midwifery Vol. 21, pp. 253–266

Independent Maternity Review (2022) Ockenden report – Final: Findings, conclusions, and essential actions from the independent review of maternity services at the Shrewsbury and Telford Hospital NHS Trust (HC 1219) Crown. Available at https://assets.publishing.service.gov.uk/government/uploads/system/uploads/attachment_data/file/1064302/Final-Ockenden-Report-web-accessible.pdf (Accessed 9th Sept 2024)

Institute for Social Capital (2025) Empowering People To Realise the Benefits and Importance of Social Relationships. Available https://www.socialcapitalresearch.com/ (Accessed 26 Jan 2025)

Kerelo S (2020) What is a professional midwifery advocate? British Journal of Midwifery 28(4):220-221

Kirkup B (2022) Reading the signals, Maternity and Neonatal Services East Kent – the report of the independent investigation. London: His Majesty's Stationary Office. Available: https://assets. publishing.service.gov.uk/media/634fb083e90e0731a5423408/reading-the-signals-maternity-and-neonatal-services-in-east-kent_the-report-of-the-independent-investigation_print-ready. pdf (accessed 28 Jan 2025)

Kirkup B (2015) The Report of the Morecambe Bay Investigation. Available: http://data.parlia-ment.uk/DepositedPapers/Files/DEP2015-0267/The_Report_of_the_Morecambe_Bay.pdf (Accessed 27 Jan 2025)

Kitson-Reynolds E (2022) Introduction. In E. Kitson-Reynolds, & K. Ashforth, (Eds) A Concise Guide to Continuity of Care in Midwifery (pp. 18–33) London and New York: Routledge

Kitson-Reynolds E and Ashforth A (2022) Ch10: Resources In E. Kitson-Reynolds, and K. Ashforth, (Eds) A Concise Guide to Continuity of Care in Midwifery (pp. 149–175) London and New York: Routledge

Kitson-Reynolds E (2020) The University of Southampton Midwifery Values Based Enquiry Journey. University of Southampton: Southampton

Lown BA, Manning CF (2010). The Schwartz center rounds: evaluation of an interdisciplinary approach to enhancing patient-centered communication, teamwork, and provider support. Acad Med. 85(6):1073–81 Available: https://doi.org/10.1097/ACM.0b013e3181dbf741 (accessed 4 Feb 2025)

Maben J, Taylor C, Dawson J, Leamy M, McCarthy I, Reynolds E, Ross S, Shuldham C, Burnett L, Foot C (2018) A realist informed mixed-methods evaluation of Schwartz Center Rounds in England. Health Serv Del Res. 37(No. 6) National Institute of Health Research.

McAra-Couper J, Gilkison A, Crowther S, Hunter M, Hotchin C, Gunn J (2014). Partnership and reciprocity with women sustain Lead Maternity Carer midwives in practice. NZCOM Journal 49, 23–33. Available: https://doi.org/10.12784/nzcomjnl49.2014.5.29-33 (accessed 24 Feb 2025)

McNeil M, Kitson-Reynolds E (2024). Student midwives' experiences of clinical placement and the decision to enter the professional register. British Journal of Midwifery 32:14-20. Available: https://www.britishjournalofmidwifery.com/content/research/student-midwives-experiences-of-clinical-placement-and-the-decision-to-enter-the-professional-register/ (accessed 26 Jan 2025)

NHS England (n.d.) A just culture guide. Available: https://www.england.nhs.uk/patient-safety/ patient-safety-culture/a-just-culture-guide/ (accessed 24 Feb 2025)

NHS England (2016) Better Births: Improving Outcomes of maternity services in England. National Maternity Review. Available at https://www.england.nhs.uk/publication/better-births-improving-outcomes-of-maternity-services-in-england-a-five-year-forward-view-for-maternity-care/ (Accessed 9 Sept 2024)

NHS England (2017) A-EQUIP midwifery supervision model. Available: https://www.england.nhs. uk/mat-transformation/implementing-better-births/a-equip/a-equip-midwifery-supervision-model/ (accessed 4 Feb 2025)

NHS England (2022) Freedom to Speak Up Policy for the NHS Available: https://www.england. nhs.uk/wp-content/uploads/2022/06/PAR1245i-NHS-freedom-to-speak-up-national-Policy-eBook.pdf (Accessed 4 Feb 2025)

NHS Leadership Academy (2025a) Regional coaching and mentoring offers. Available: https:// www.leadershipacademy.nhs.uk/programmes/coaching-and-mentoring/regional-coaching-and-mentoring-offers/ (assessed 18 Jan 2025)

NHS England (2025) Culture and Leadership Programme. Available: https://www.england.nhs.uk/ culture/culture-leadership-programme/#:~:text=The%20Culture%20and%20Leadership%20 Programme%20provides%20a%20practical%2C%20evidence%2Dbased,on%20 our%20online%20learning%20page. (Accessed 26 Jan 2025)

NHS Education Scotland (2025) Leading for the Future. Available: https://learn.nes.nhs.scot/18217/leadership-and-management-programmes#:~:text=Leading%20for%20the%20Future,Leadership%20Foundations (accessed 26 Jan 2025).

NHS Leadership Academy (2025b) NHS Leadership Academy. https://www.leadershipacademy.nhs.uk (assessed 18 January 2025)

Nursing and Midwifery Council (2019) Standards for Pre-registration Midwifery Programmes. Nursing and Midwifery Council, London. Available: https://www.nmc.org.uk/globalassets/sitedocuments/standards/2024/standards-of-proficiency-for-midwives.pdf (Accessed 24 Feb 2025)

Maben J, Taylor C, Jagosh J, Carrieri D, Briscoe S, Klepacz N, Mattick K (2023) Delivering healthcare: a complex balancing act: A guide to understanding and tackling psychological ill-health in nurses, midwives and paramedics. University of Surrey, Guildford. www.workforceresearchsurrey.health

O'Brien M (2022) Case load practice and the national and international political/professional context. In E. Kitson-Reynolds, & K. Ashforth, (Eds) A Concise Guide to Continuity of Care in Midwifery (pp. 18–33) London and New York: Routledge

O'Brien M (2018b) Respectful Relationships in Maternity Services. Presentation presented at the Northern Maternity and Midwifery Festival. Manchester. 26 June 2018

O'Brien M (2018c) Practical Steps to Developing a Respectful and Caring Workplace: Challenging Bullying Behaviours. Cardiff. 20 Sept 2018

Oxford English Dictionary (2025) Oxford University Press. Oxford Available at: https://www.oxfordlearnersdictionaries.com/definition/english/golden-thread?q=golden+thread (Accessed 28 Feb 2025)

Point of Care Foundation (2015) Schwartz Rounds. Available: http://www.pointofcarefoundation.org.uk/our-work/Schwartz-rounds/ (accessed 4 Feb 2025)

Riley G, Aldridge P, Taylor-Anjous N, Roseveare S (2023). Evaluation Summary of the Black Maternity Matters Pilot. West of England Academic Health Science Network. Available: https://www.healthinnowest.net/wp-content/uploads/2023/03/Black-Maternity-Matters-Evaluation-Summary-February-2023.pdf (accessed 25 Feb 2025).

Royal College Midwives (2016) Why midwives leave—revisited. RCM, London, England Available: https://cdn.ps.emapcom/wp-content/uploads/sites/3/2016/10/Why-Midwives-Leave (accessed 26 Jan 2025)

Royal College Midwives (2017) Findings of the RCM Survey of the Health, Safety and Wellbeing of Midwives and Maternity Support Workers Available: https://rcm.org.uk/wp-content/uploads/2024/06/caring-for-you-evaluation-findings-of-the-rcm-s-survey-of-the-health-safety-and-wellbeing-of-midwives-and-maternity-support-workers.pdf (accessed 24 Feb 2025)

Royal College of Midwives (2025) RCM Available at: https://rcm.org.uk/ (Accessed 31 Jan 2025)

Royal College of Nursing (2025) RCN the voice of nursing. Available at: https://www.rcn.org.uk/ (Accessed 31 Jan 2025)

Sedgewick-Müller J (2024) Supporting students living with ADHD at university: working better together. Takeda, UK

Smith J (2021) Nurturing Maternity Staff. How to tackle trauma, stress and burnout to create a positive working culture in the NHS. Pinter and Martin, London

Trades Union Congress (2025) TUC, Changing the world of work for good. Available: https://www.tuc.org.uk/ (Accessed 31 Jan 2025)

UNISON (2025) UNISON the public service union. Available at https://www.unison.org.uk/about/what-we-do/ (accessed 31 Jan 2025)

West M, Bailey S, Williams E (2020) The courage of compassion: supporting nurses and midwives to deliver high-quality care. Kings Fund /RCN Foundation, London Available: https://www.kingsfund.org.uk/insight-and-analysis/reports/courage-compassion-supporting-nurses-midwives (Accessed 4 Feb 2025)

West MA (2021) Leadership self-compassion. MA West (Ed) Compassionate Leadership: Sustaining Wisdom, Humanity and Presence Health and Social Care. (pp. 207–224) London: Swirling Leaf Press.

West M, Eckert R, Collins B, Chowla R, (2017) Caring to change: how compassionate leadership can stimulate innovation in health care 2017. The Kings Fund Available: https://assets.kings-fund.org.uk/f/256914/x/0b76247d02/caring_to_change_2017.pdf (Accessed 24 Feb 2025)

Whitmore J (2009) Coaching for Performance: GROWing Human Potential and Purpose. The Principles and Practice of Coaching Leadership, 4 Edn. Nicholas Brealey Publishing, London; Boston

Wilson C, Hall L, Chilvers R (2018) Where are the consultant midwives? BJM 26(4) Available: https://www.britishjournalofmidwifery.com/content/professional/where-are-the-consultant-midwives/ (Accessed 4 Feb 2025)

Wylam (2023) Why do Newly Qualified and Student Midwives Leave. In A Barrett, A Burleigh, P Gillen, D Hughes (Eds.) #saynotobullyinginmidwifery (pp 116–199). Available: www.mid-wifery.org.uk/news/support/saynotobullyinginmidwifery-report/ (accessed 26 Jan 2025)

# Correction to: Respectful Relationships in the Maternity Service

Maggie O'Brien and Ellen Kitson-Reynolds

---

**Correction to:**
**M. O'Brien, E. Kitson-Reynolds (eds.), *Respectful Relationships in the Maternity Service*,**
**https://doi.org/10.1007/978-3-032-04281-1**

The book was inadvertently published without the Index. This has been included in the corrected version.

---

The updated version of this book can be found at
https://doi.org/10.1007/978-3-032-04281-1


M. O'Brien, E. Kitson-Reynolds (eds.), *Respectful Relationships in the Maternity
Service*, https://doi.org/10.1007/978-3-032-04281-1_9

# Index

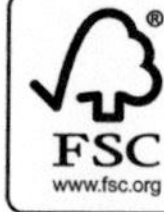

MIX
Papier aus verantwortungsvollen Quellen
Paper from responsible sources
FSC® C105338

If you have any concerns about our products,
you can contact us on
ProductSafety@springernature.com

In case Publisher is established outside the EU,
the EU authorized representative is:
**Springer Nature Customer Service Center GmbH**
**Europaplatz 3, 69115 Heidelberg, Germany**

Printed by Libri Plureos GmbH
in Hamburg, Germany